D1653952

Yoga RX for the 12 Steps

▪▪▪▪▪▪▪▪▪▪▪▪▪ Simone King

Photos by David Papas

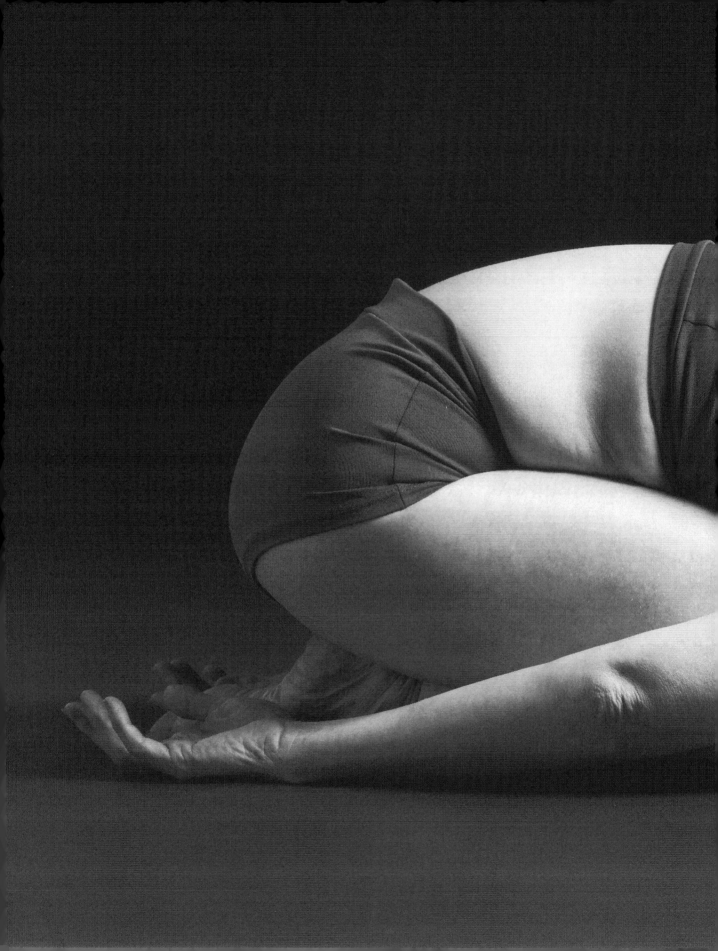

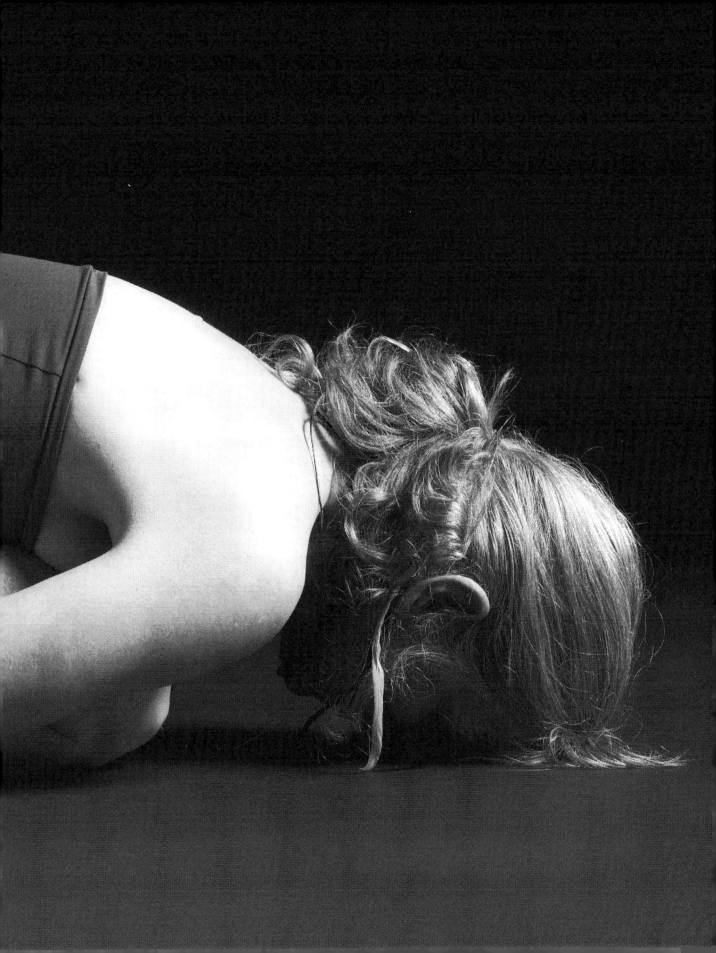

2011
Left Eye of the Bird
555 12th Street, Suite 1440
Oakland, CA 94607

Copyright 2011 Left Eye of the Bird
Text copyright 2011 Simone King

All right reserved. No part of this book may
be reproduced by any means or in any other form
whatsoever without written permission from the
publisher, except for brief quotations embodied in
literary articles or reviews.

Printed in the United States of America

ISBN-13: 978-1466416024
ISBN-10: 146641605

Book and Cover Design:
Adriana Fracchia

Special thanks to the models:
Justin Petallero, Jackie Cheng,
Jennifer Schmitt, John Kidder
and Ezra King

Dedicated to my teachers:

Bikram Choudhry, Mark Whilwell, and most of all, Daniel King. He was the only person in my life who looked at me and said, "You're amazing, I love you, and if you drink I want nothing to do with you." He not only provided the spark that saved my life, he showed me a way of being in the world. We dated by going to Bikram yoga and had 17 beautiful years. Daniel died in 2003, but together we had three wonderful sons, Elijah, Aidan and Ezra. They continue to teach me more about love and life than I ever thought possible.

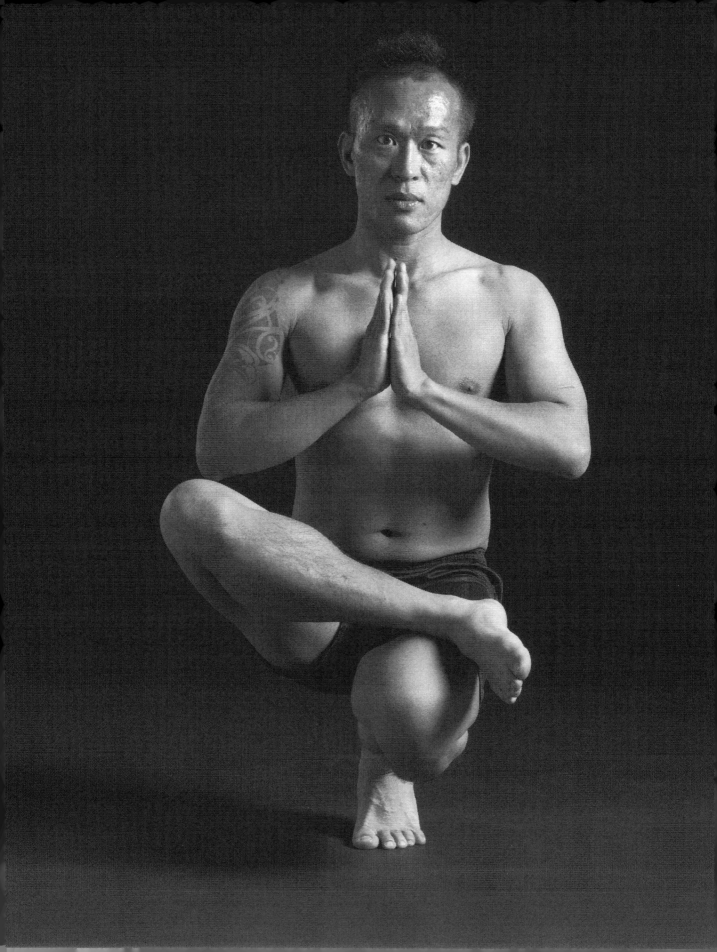

The descent to Hell is easy.
But to make one's way, to retrace
the steps up, out into the golden air
That is difficult,
             -and this is the work.

Virgil

TABLE OF CONTENTS

Foreword by Mark Whitwell	1
Introduction	6
Why Yoga?	12
Why Include Partner Postures?	18
Breathing	22

The Postures

STEP ONE:	Bound Angle Pose	29
	Fixed Firm	31
	Child / Fish	33
STEP TWO:	Triangle	37
	Standing Backward Bend	39
	Massage Table	41
STEP THREE:	Half Tortoise	45
	Standing Head to Knee	47
	Hanging Lift	49
STEP FOUR:	Warrior I	53
	Chair	55
	Breathe With Me	57
STEP FIVE:	Lion	63
	Standing Bow	65
	Backpack	67
STEP SIX:	Spinal Twist	71
	Shoulder Stand	Plough	73
	Assisted Handstand	75

TABLE OF CONTENTS (continued)

STEP SEVEN:	Downward Dog	79
	Camel	81
	Honoring	83
STEP EIGHT:	Rabbit	87
	Tiger	89
	Double Tree / Lean on Me	91
STEP NINE:	Balancing Stick	97
	Pigeon	99
	Standing Twist	101
STEP TEN:	Tree	105
	Eagle	107
	Double Triangle	109
STEP ELEVEN:	Savasana	115
	Lotus	117
	Double Savasana	119
	Double Lotus	
STEP TWELVE:	Bridge	124
	Wheel	125
	Falcon	129

Flows

Flow I: Anxiety	135
Flow II: Depression	137
Flow III: Insomnia	139
Recommended Reading List	142
Index	146

FORWARD | MARK WHITWELL

I have seen Simone's transformation. She has taught me so much. She showed me just how bad addiction can get. I was shocked to see my friend pulled down physically, emotionally and spiritually. I was frightened to see the grip addiction had taken. It seemed impossible to turn the degradation around. Then she showed me the power of yoga practice.

Simone is a friend whom I love. As her friend and teacher, I was able to intervene in her life. The daily circumstances were devastating. The light in her seemed to have completely gone out. I gave her a short, daily yoga practice that was right for her. I know that yoga is each person's direct intimacy with Reality, which is nothing other than Nurturing Source. Through my insistence, Simone made "The Promise" and took the first step. Immediately, the force of Life, the healing power of nurturing source intrinsic to life, kicked in. She began to look and feel better! She became less despondent and no longer dependent on intoxication. Something else was bringing her pleasure on a daily basis. As time went by, I witnessed Simone become a whole person. She was totally present, fully functioning in the extreme intelligence and beauty that is Life. She has developed a profound relationship to herself, the people she touches and to Nurturing Source. Today I know a happy person, a fully expressed woman, mother, teacher and lover. I see a person you can trust to teach you your Yoga. That is not just any yoga, but YOUR Yoga. It is your direct intimacy with life! Please listen to this person. She has seen it all, from high to low, low to high. These are the people who make the best kinds of teachers. They are the "acharya," those who have overcome their own restrictions. They know the process by which this is possible and are able to show others how to overcome too!

–With Love and Gratitude, Mark Whitwell
Author, *Yoga of Heart* and *The Promise*

STRETCHING SOUND is **MUSIC**

STRETCHING MOVEMENT is **DANCE**

STRETCHING the SMILE is **LAUGHTER**

STRETCHING the MIND is **MEDITATION**

STRETCHING the DEVOTEE is **GOD**

STRETCHING FEELING is **ECSTASY**

STRETCHING EMPTINESS is **BLISS**

INTRODUCTION

He put his trust in a Higher Power

He held his power like a Holy Grail

He summoned all of his faith in the lifting

He suffered all of his faith if he failed

His heart was stronger than a heavy metal bullet...

He was a good man and now he's gone

–M. Ward

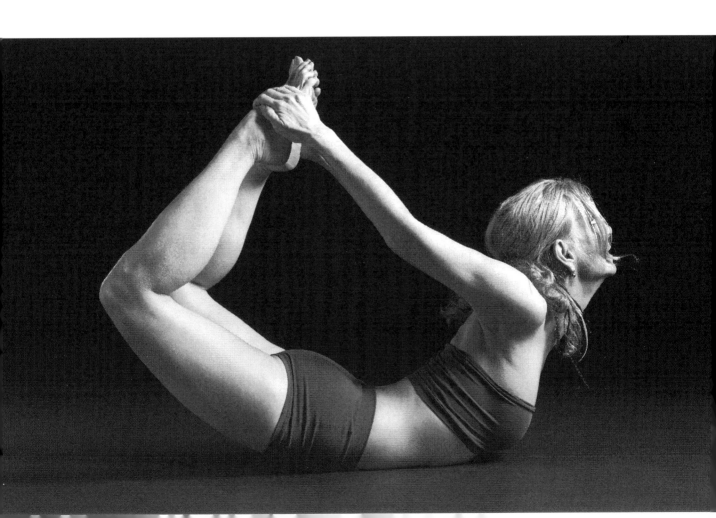

INTRODUCTION (continued)

I don't conceive of my addiction as a heavy metal bullet, although I can find truth in that analogy. Addiction definitely causes me to face my mortality on a daily basis. My favorite quote is from the NA literature when they state the final outcome will be, "Jails, institutions, and death." I realize the only way for me to avert these inevitable outcomes is to walk in faith and pray for grace.

For me, addiction is a demon that lives, asleep in my brain. If I do all the right things, it will stay asleep. If it wakes up, I am in serious trouble. Its waking can come from many things: stress, loneliness, anger, and of course, drinking. Once it's awake, I don't stand a chance. It wants me dead. Actually, the demon only wants alcohol. My death, incarceration or institutional commitment would be collateral damage. They would be by products of the demon's desire to drink.

Going to meetings, having a sponsor, working the steps and helping others are the things that keep my demon asleep. Also high on that list is practicing yoga. Yoga helps to keep the stress, loneliness, and fear at bay. It works on the physical, mental, emotional, energetic, and spiritual bodies. Regular practice can be enormously helpful in implementing a twelve step program of recovery.

Recovery is ultimately a spiritual program. My teacher Mark Whitwell says, "Yoga is a technology for creating conscious contact with God." When practiced regularly, it creates a direct link to one's Higher Power. You can substitute Cosmic Consciousness, the Universe, Allah, Prana, Qi, Odin or a doorknob. Whatever terminology works for you.

Many people are intimidated by yoga. It is a discipline. Since it works on so many levels, it can be physically, mentally, emotionally and spiritually challenging. However, as another one of my teacher's states, "Yoga meets you where you are at and moves you in a positive direction." In the Bhagavad Gita, Krishna tells Arjuna, "Even the abortive attempt is not wasted. Nor can it produce contrary results. Even a little practice of yoga will save you from the terrible wheel of life and death." Doing asana and pranayama, moving and breathing, are all it takes to garner many benefits. It is a practice. All that is required is sincere effort. The results are automatic.

A therapist once referred to my son as, "A nervous critter." I suffer from the same affliction. I have been traumatized repeatedly. My drinking stemmed from the desire to be sedated. Yoga treats this condition for me. Practicing regularly allows my nervous system to calm down. In the beginning, stretching and breathing allowed me to sit still through a meeting. Eventually, following the directions of a teacher in class allowed me to practice doing what I was told. This translated in to being able to accept direction from my sponsor and other people in recovery. Improving balance and alignment, creating mental focus by finding somewhere to put my brain, these benefits of yoga practice have allowed me to venture in to recovery and to grow along the 12 step path. The asana serves the breath and the breath embodies recovery.

There is a growing body of empirical evidence to support these assertions. In an *L.A. Times* article dated 17 Aug. 2010, it states, "Available review of a wide range of yoga practices suggest they can reduce the impact of exaggerated stress response and may be helpful for both anxiety and depression. By reducing perceived stress and anxiety, yoga appears to modulate the stress response system. This, in turn, decreases physiological arousal. For example, decreased heart rate, lower blood pressure and increased ease of respiration. There is also evidence that yoga practice helps increase heart rate variability, an indicator of the body's ability to respond to stress more flexibly."

Simply put, this is something I say in every class: "You are reprogramming your nervous

INTRODUCTION (continued)

system. You are training your body to respond differently to stress. By practicing the postures and linking them to your breath, you are teaching yourself to relax on command. We do postures that jack your heart rate up, then teach you to use your breath to bring your heart rate down. It is marriage of the heart and lungs, marriage of the mind and body, marriage of body and breath."

Yoga is good medicine. It is possible to prescribe particular postures to address whatever is limiting someone. This book provides prescriptions for working each of the twelve steps. In the back are flows designed to address depression, insomnia, and anxiety. These three problems seem to plague most people, especially in early recovery. The book is designed for everyone, from experienced practitioners to people who have never tried yoga. Just do your best and remember to breathe.

I began my Bikram yoga practice in 1986. I got into recovery in 1988. The latter would not have been possible without the former. Yoga taught me to breathe, to be still and to accept direction from another human being. In recovery, I have survived many experiences, good and bad: A happy marriage, the sudden death of my husband, giving birth to beautiful children, having a son choose to live on the streets, economic abundance and economic apocalypse. Through all of this, yoga has sustained and guided me. I hope it is helpful to you. I am curious to hear how it goes.

If you have questions, comments, criticisms, please let me know. You can e mail me at Simone@LETB.ME. I look forward to hearing from you.

WHY YOGA?

The Yoga sutras suggest we deliberately turn away from the choice for death and embrace the choice for Life.

Yoga is an exercise for creating spiritual fitness. Ultimately, recovery is a spiritual program. When I first got sober, people in AA would talk about being spiritually fit. I had no concept of what that could possibly mean. I have come to understand this term to refer to a state of being aligned with a higher power so that information and guidance flow freely. Serenity is a product of spiritual fitness. Being spiritually fit requires action. Yoga is an exercise that generates spiritual fitness. It is a moving meditation, a technology for creating conscious contact with God.

yoga is an **exercise** for creating **spiritual fitness**

> *Telling an addict who is freaking out to calm down does no good. The world of the addict is a crazy world, but it is home. The world of a recovering addict is a different crazy. It is a foreign crazy for which there are no emotional coping mechanisms.*
>
> —Bucky Sinister, *Get Up*

Yoga can provide a road map for developing emotional coping mechanisms.

> *When you practice yoga, constrictions around the heart fall away. The first insight of yoga is said to be that you know your heart is restricted. It may make you feel vulnerability to know this, but there is power in this vulnerability because it is honest. Being close to the truth is being close to the power of life. Yoga is what you can do in the midst of feeling restricted. It is your direct connection to Truth. Find your depths at your heart.*

WHY YOGA (continued)

By participating in your whole body, you realize life's energy and intelligence. The culminating point of the fullness of feeling is the heart, the hrid, the seat of the mind and body, the portal between spirit and form.

–Mark Whitwell, *Yoga of Heart*

yoga can provide a **road map** for developing **emotional coping mechanisms**

The word for the heart in ancient Sanskrit is Hridaya. Hri means to give, and daya is to receive. The practice of yoga teaches your being to give and receive in a sacred, therefore spiritual, therefore safe and healthy way.

Learning how to do this has been essential for my recovery. The family I grew up in left me with no model for relating to people. Everything I learned at home was repellant. I knew what I did not want to be, but had no idea of what I wanted, and less of a clue on how to get there. I was lucky. I was given the gift of yoga which provided a blueprint for my body and a technology for my mind. I learned to discipline my mind by focusing on the body and developed the ability to use my breath mindfully, with control.

I am increasingly convinced that the power of yoga is unleashed by getting the mind to inhabit the body. When you know your whole body, you can realize the heart. Anyone who arrives at 12 Step recovery has experienced trauma, either as the result of their addiction or from life experiences. Often there are family of origin issues that have encouraged the mind to flee from physical experience. For a person with a history of physical trauma, the body is a dangerous place to be. In Somatic Psychology they say that every person's experience is stored in the body. Your history is present in the memory of the muscles and membranes. Dealing with the wreckage of the past is a large part of the work of a 12 Step program of recovery. By incorporating the practice of yoga into working the steps you can take this work all the way from the level of your cells to your spirit.

> *I thought recovery was a way to get out of myself, like I tried to do with drugs & alcohol. The words of the third step prayer are "to be relieved of the bondage of self." I have come to understand that the tools of recovery help me turn my body from a prison into a playground. But I have to stay home to do this.*
>
> —Guy at my Sunday Morning Meeting

He could just as well have been talking about yoga. Yoga helps people develop a sense of ease, a sense of comfort and a sense of presence, inside their bodies and inside their minds. Recovery and yoga together is a powerful combination to help you move out of prison and into playfulness.

I can take my mind and put it in the corner of the room. I used to think this was an awesome coping mechanism. When I needed it, it was. It allowed me to survive. When I got sober, I learned that this ability has a psychiatric definition. It is called dissociation.

The dissociative response is common among people who have been traumatized. The mind needs to escape because the body is too painful of a place to be. Yoga has allowed me to reintegrate my mind with my body. Yoga directly combats the effects of trauma in the body. With trauma the mind is constantly on high alert. Most people experience a state of hyper vigilance. They are continuously scanning the environment for signs of impending danger. In the body this chronically triggers the sympathetic nervous response, commonly referred to as fight or flight.

WHY YOGA (continued)

The physiological effects of the chronic stress response include:

- Release of epinephrine (adrenaline), norepinephrine & dopamine
- Increased heart rate and strength of contraction
- Increased blood pressure
- Increased respiratory rate
- Increased blood flow to skeletal muscles
- Inhibition of digestive functions

By practicing yoga, you can train your body to relax on command. When you calm the body down, it relaxes the mind. It is a two way street. By closing your mouth, breathing long and slow and deep through your nose, you trigger the parasympathetic response. This directly counter acts the effects of stress and trauma. The parasympathetic is responsible for stimulating the activities that occur when the body is at rest.

I began drinking at age ten and drank alcoholically by the time I was twelve. It is difficult to imagine the damage I did to my developing brain and nervous system. Some people contend this damage is irreversible. I happen to believe my brain, body, and being have found alternate pathways, mostly through the practice of yoga. I know as a fact that moving and breathing, learning to focus and meditate have allowed me to counteract some of the most damaging effects of my early and extensive drinking.

Despite the catchy title, the postures in the book are suggested as being helpful to a program of recovery. To bring this together I started by interviewing over 100 people in 12 step recovery programs. I asked them to describe each step with one or two words. I compiled the responses and distilled them down to the terms which came up most often and were most inclusive. I then prescribed postures out of my own practice and experience. These postures will not appeal to everyone, although they should be accessible and effective for most.

I won't say all yoga is good yoga. However, I do believe that more yoga is good, and that there is a yoga style or teacher for each and every student. I often say that yoga is like ice cream. I happen to like pistachio. Not everyone does. But if you keep looking, keep trying samples, you will find a flavor of yoga practice that works for you. If you try something and hate it, move on. Ask for samples. It is trial and error, but where a sincere desire to learn exist, the teacher will appear. The idea I hope readers take away from this text is that a regular, personal yoga practice is an invaluable asset to working a program of recovery. This book is a good place to start. I've included a Recommended Reading List at the back. Do a little research. Ask people you know who have a practice that works for them. Get over the fear, or ego, or inflexibility that keeps you from trying. Yoga has become very popular. The current incarnations of thousands of years of wisdom culture are more available and accessible than every before. Make use of this powerful resource and enjoy.

WHY INCLUDE PARTNER POSES?

> *Sharing the life force is what brings people together;
> with it, love and compassion naturally flow.*
>
> –Bruce Frantzis

> *If you imagine yourself to be separate from others you are in pain.
> There is no God realization in isolation.*
>
> –Mark Whitwell

We all want to feel more connected. In recovery it is essential. It is impossible to recover alone. You have to reach out to other human beings. Unfortunately, many of us don't know how to do this. Or we learned "how" by copying what we saw around us. No one really teaches us how to relate. What we see is a skewed version of relating embedded in a society that has a skewed relationship to touch.

Our society is touch negative. Touch is either avoided or sexualized. Sex is then packaged and objectified. It is used to sell everything from razor blades to milk to car insurance. Yet somehow it remains covert, dirty and sometimes shameful. It is very confusing, not to mention dysfunctional and discouraging. The result is we touch each other less and less.

Partner yoga is a simple tool to learn to be comfortable, relaxed and at ease while directly

WHY INCLUDE PARTNER POSES (continued)

interacting with another person. It allows you to safely explore touch. Using the breath, you learn to open your heart to someone else. You are then able to create more intimate connections. As you open your heart, your partner works on opening theirs. You can feel the life force, the prana, move between the two of you. If you allow yourself to receive this, the relationship will begin to shift. Partner yoga meets any relationship where it exists in the present and moves it in a positive direction.

You also get to practice other elements of successful relationship in a safe arena. The roles are clearly defined, the goals are clear and limited. Partner yoga requires direct communication with terms agreed upon beforehand. To perform partner postures safely, you have to listen to each other. Sometimes you have to mirror one another. It is essential to tune in to your partner and stay focused. Sometimes you have to trust your partner. Sometimes you have to support your partner. You always have to be present for one another. There is a visceral feeling of connection. You feel connected and begin to embody that fully. As you practice partner yoga, you begin to feel a stronger and deeper connection to the Source of Life, to your partner and to Love. Restrictions will fall away from your heart. These are tools to help you navigate relationship consciously. You are creating the possibility of feeling grace, peace, power and beauty with everyone in your life.

BREATHING

Yoga means union, marriage, a yoking together. The vehicle that creates union is breath. The breath links the heart and lungs, mind and body, being and God.

Asana (posture) serves the Breath, and the Breath serves God.

In yoga, your breath must initiate each gesture and envelopes your movement. You begin to breathe slightly before moving and continue to breathe slightly after the movement ends.

It is essential to link the movement with the breath. This brings awareness into your body. In many texts, prana, life energy, is translated from Sanskrit as breath. When you move the breath you are also moving your energy, mingling it with the energy of life and engaging with that which is greater than all of us.

asana (posture) serves the breath, and the breath serves god

When I work with people I talk a lot about moving energy. I often tell them, "Learn to run your energy instead of letting your energy run you." As a practicing alcoholic, my unrestrained energy will drive me deeper into addiction. There is a part of my nature that is bent on destruction. Learning to harness this energy and direct it in a positive flow not only opens me up to all of life, it helps keep me from running headlong towards certain death.

When the movement and breath are linked, yoga helps you create an intimate relationship with your own body. You develop intimacy with your body through using the breath to bring awareness (mind) into specific places and exploring your internal experience. You breathe, relax and get to know yourself from the inside out.

Breathing (continued)

PRANAYAMA

Pranayam is a Sanskrit word meaning, "restraint of the prana or life force." The English dictionary defines pranayama as "a type of yogic breath awareness and regulation exercise designed to help control one's vital energy." There are hundreds of these exercises. Here are a few simple ones that can have powerful results if practiced regularly.

DEEP BREATHING

Sometimes this technique is referred to as Belly Breathing. When my sons were young, I taught them to get their belly buttons to breath. This dropped their awareness down to their bellies and automatically caused them to breathe more slowly and deeply.

A more sophisticated way to practice is to place one hand on the chest and one on the lower belly. Inhale, taking a long slow deep breath. Pull the air to the back of the nose. Fill the lungs to capacity and allow the belly rise as the lungs inflate. Then let the air to go out of the lungs and feel the belly fall with the exhale. Do this for a few breaths then start to actively exhale, contracting the abdominal muscles to push the air out of the lungs.

The benefits of deep breathing include: increased lung capacity, increased gas exchange leading to more oxygen in, more toxins out, and increased metabolism due to more oxygen getting to the tissues. It also tones abdominal muscles, and calms and focuses the mind. Nitric oxide is released in the nasal cavity. Nitric oxide is a vasodilator, increasing blood flow. It also potentiates the action of dopamine and seratonin in the synapses of the nerves.

Deep breathing activates a relaxation response on a physiological level. An important mechanism of the relaxation response is mediated via the vagus nerve. The neurotransmitter used by the parasympathetic nervous system is acetylcholine. The brain connects to the diaphragm through the release of acetylcholine from the vagus nerve.

Acetylcholine also plays and important role in learning and the formation of memory. New research indicates that the release of acetylcholine calms down the inflammatory response in the body. This is particularly exciting news for the millions of people suffering from autoimmune diseases. Another promising area of current research is establishing a link between activation of the vagus nerve and cellular regeneration both in the tissues of the brain and in the production of stem cells throughout the body.

Stimulation of the vagus nerve leads to increased feelings of peace and relaxation, increased potential for learning and memory, decreased inflammation and increased cell regeneration and repair.

How do you stimulate the vagus nerve? You can activate all these benefits by breathing long and slow and deep. When you take a deep breath, the movement of the diaphragm massages the vagus nerve. This releases acetylcholine and activates the parasympathetic (relaxation) response.

RHYTHMIC BREATHING

With rhythmic breathing, you elongate the exhale. Breathe in for a count of four and breathe out for a count of eight. Or, breath in for three and out for six. The numbers do not matter, it is the ratio that is important. If you have trouble with this you can try inhale, pause, exhale. You lose the effects of extended exhale but some people find this more accessible.

The benefits of rhythmic breathing are dramatic. Prolonged exhale activates the parasympathetic nervous system, engaging the actions of the body at rest. It lowers heart rate, calms the mind and relaxes skeletal muscles. You are also working to purify the body by releasing more toxins as the length of exhale increases. A longer exhale creates potential for greater gas exchange by increasing the vacuum effect so the following inhale is stronger.

Breathing (continued)

ALTERNATE NOSTRIL BREATHING

Close your right nostril with your right thumb. Let the rest of your fingers point to the top of your head. Inhale through the left nostril. Close the left nostril with the right pinkie. Exhale through the right nostril. Inhale right and close. Exhale left, this equals one cycle. Repeat for ten cycles.

Benefits of Alternate Nostril Breathing: It balances left and right hemispheres of the brain, helps brain integrate information, alleviates headaches, regulates heating and cooling cycles of the body, and promotes deep relaxation.

STEP ONE

Powerlessness & Surrender

- Bound Angle
- Fixed Firm
- Child / Fish

"We admitted we were powerless over alcohol—that our lives had become unmanageable."

Bound Angle Pose *Baddha Konasana*

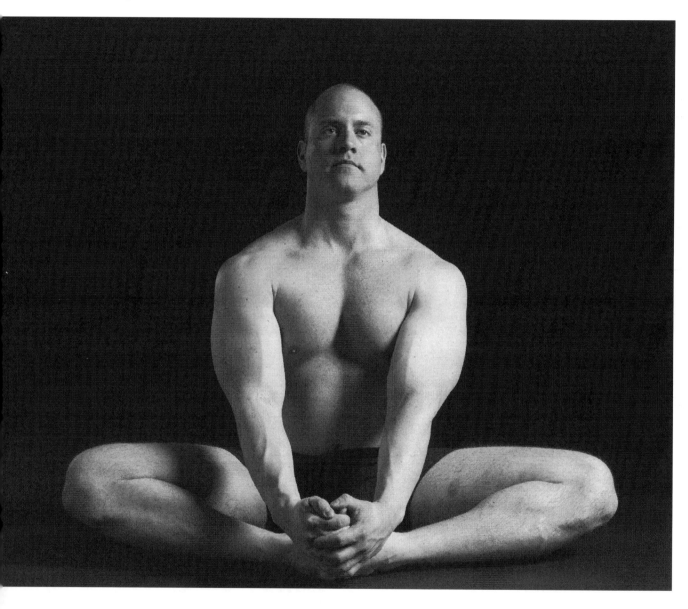

Bound Angle enables us to embody the First Step, to experience it on a physical level. Admitting we are powerless can feel like being in a bind. You declare there is a huge problem AND recognize that there is nothing you can do about it. Practicing Baddha Konasana can give physical representation to this feeling of being in a bind. It is both an acknowledgement and a path through. By breathing and relaxing, the feeling of stricture can diminish as the student deepens into the pose. Eventually there is a comfort in the posture, ultimately bowing the head in an act of surrender.

Sit facing forward, knees bent and feet flat on the floor. Slide the heels toward the pelvis, allowing the knees to fall to the side. Bring the soles of the feet to touch. Place hands on feet or shins. The goal is to get knees to the floor. Once the knees touch the floor, begin moving the heels closer to the pelvis. Final expression is to bow the head and touch forehead to feet.

Physical Benefits

- Stretches inner thighs, groin and knees
- Stimulates abdominal organs
- Good for flat feet

Fixed Firm *Supta Vajrasana*

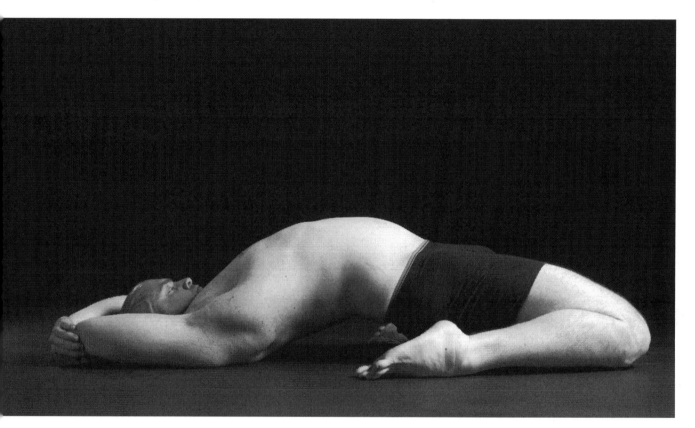

Swimmers who fight against the water tire and drown.

Those who relax into it, float.

Step One

Progress in this posture is incremental. Do not push your knees too far. Go to a level of discomfort you can tolerate and STAY there. The body's natural response to pain is to resist and avoid. When something hurts or you feel fear, the muscles contract and clench. By learning how to relax into the resistance, you are working on reprogramming your relationship to pain. To soften instead of tighten, move toward instead of avoid, is a revolutionary act. Increasing one's tolerance comes as the body softens and the breath moves into areas that are constricted. In its final expression the posture has the feeling of complete surrender with the heart wide open. See if you can ease into, and find comfort, in a place of powerlessness and vulnerability.

Sit, knees together, feet together, hips on heels. Open heels wide enough to snuggle hips down between the heels. You can separate your knees as wide as you need to do so. You want heels touching the hips and hips on the floor. This is the first goal. Pay close attention to your knees and stop just before anything really hurts. A little discomfort is good, but being able to sustain in the posture is also important. If you can tolerate the first position, place your hands on your heels and go back one elbow at a time. Eventually you get your whole upper back on the floor. Then raise the arms overhead and grab elbows. Lift your chest up toward the ceiling. If you can do all this, start working your knees back together, making sure they do not pop up off the ground.

Physical Benefits

- Increases blood flow to knees and ankles
- Improves flexibility of hips, knees and ankles
- Increases pain tolerance

Child / Fish *Half Tortoise / Fish*

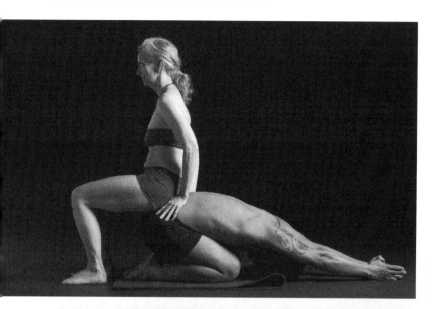
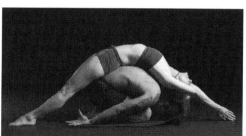
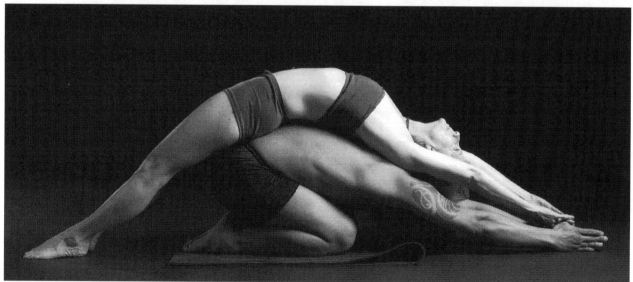

Physical Benefits

PARTNER 1
- Lengthens spine
- Stretches hips
- Releases muscles in lower back

PARTNER 2
- Opens chest, throat, shoulders
- Expands rib cage
- Releases stagnant energy from area around heart

Partner 1 gets the restorative benefits of child or half tortoise with the added security and strength of feeling their partner resting across the broadness of the back. Partner 2 exercises trust and release as they blindly relax onto the stability of their partner. Partner 1 experiences surrender to what is, literally, a higher power, the weight of Partner 2. Child and Half Tortoise are grounded, secure postures, so this surrender is experienced in a place of security, comfort and strength. Partner 2 is able to completely give all the body weight over to someone else, another form of surrender, requiring the exercise of trust.

Partner 1 kneels on mat in either child pose or half tortoise. Partner 2 sits squarely on Partner 1's hips. Partner 2 brings arms over head and reclines back across Partner 1's back. At the same time Partner 2 extends legs out in front, releasing all the weight onto Partner 1's back. Partner 2 can bring arms down along side, or both partners can extend arms out straight and hold hands. Partner 2 then expands the chest, opens the heart and relaxes.

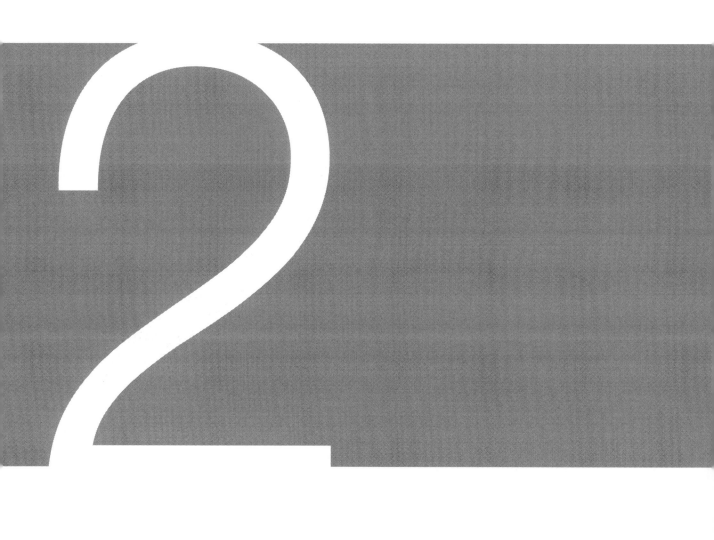

STEP TWO

Hope, Faith, & Belief

- **Triangle**
- **Backbend**
- **Massage Table**

"Came to believe that a Power greater than ourselves could restore us to sanity."

Triangle *Trikonasana*

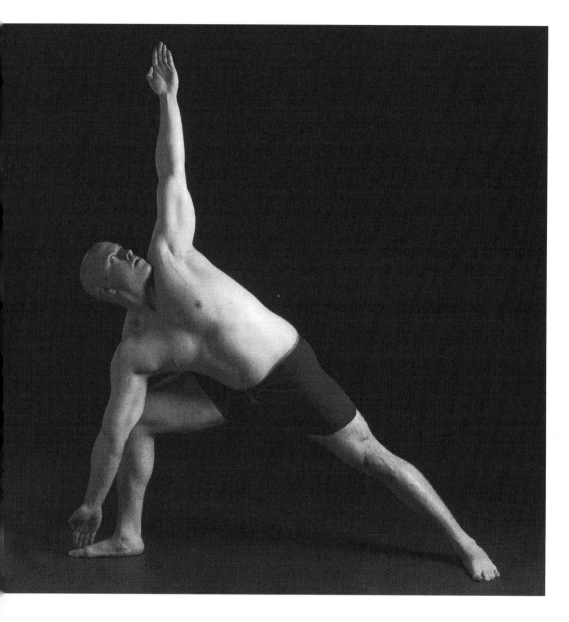

Physical Benefits

- Increases strength and flexibility of the hip joint
- Firms upper thighs and hips, slims waist
- Opens chest
- Revitalizes nerves

When done correctly and practiced regularly, Triangle opens up the area at the top of the spine, base of the skull. Yogis refer to this area as the, "mouth of God." For me, it creates direct connection with my Higher Power. I use imagery from the first *Matrix* movie where they have plugs in the backs of their head. Yoga is a technology for creating conscious contact with a higher power. Triangle offers the opportunity to plug directly in to cosmic consciousness.

Separate the legs four feet. Keeping heels aligned, turn the right foot to the right so it is perpendicular. Extend the arms straight out from the shoulders. Tighten all the muscles in the arms. Bend the right knee and drop the hips down until the right thigh is parallel to the floor. Make sure the right knee is directly over the right foot. Try to keep the spine straight in the center. Pivot the upper body so the right elbow is pressing against the right knee. The right finger tips brush the right toes. Do not put any weight on that hand or arm. The left arm extends up to the ceiling. Bring your chin to your left shoulder. Upper body is twisting. Energy in this posture is going up. The gaze is past the fingers, through the ceiling to the sky. Hold here and breathe. Reverse the process and repeat on left side.

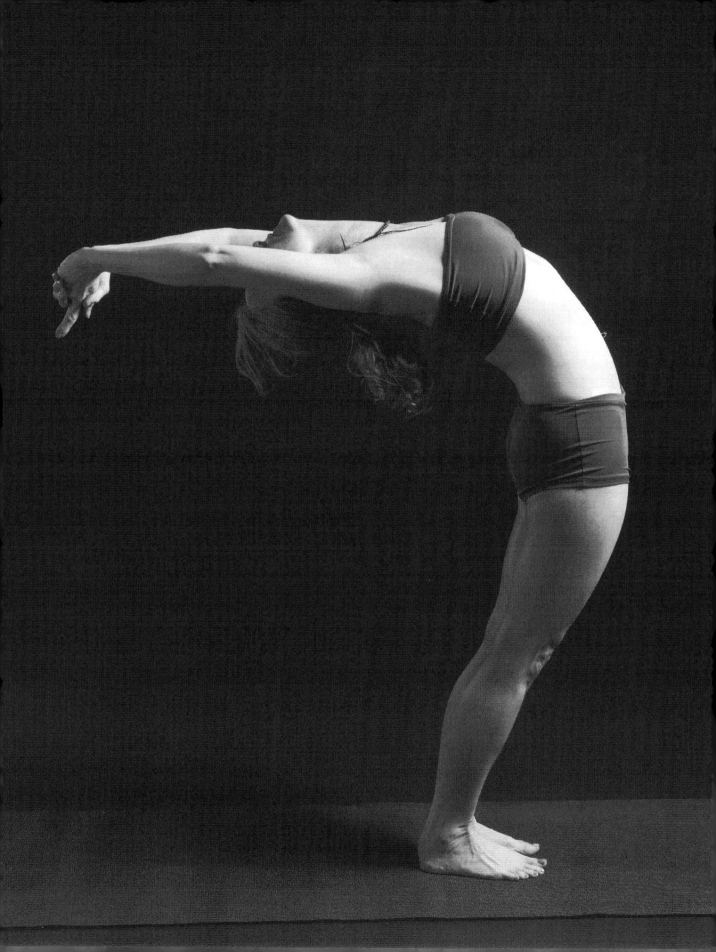

Physical Benefits

- Opens chest, shoulders
- Firms buttocks, back of thighs
- Increases flexibility of the spine

Standing Backward Bend

Backbends scare people. It takes a degree of trust, in oneself or one's teacher to release the neck and drop the head back. After all, you cannot see where you are going. It is blind movement into unknown territory. It is a position in which you are completely vulnerable. This can be emotionally intense. The key is to relax, breathe and take that leap of faith, knowing you are going to be okay. If done mindfully, there is very little risk of injury. Facing the fear of moving blindly into the unknown requires that one learns the technique and begins to trust the process. By doing so you are able to access the many healing benefits of backward bending. This makes back bends an ideal practice for people working on developing the faith necessary to work Step Two.

Stand with the feet together. Inhale and extend arms overhead. As you exhale release your neck muscles and relax your head back as far as it goes. Begin pushing your hips and pelvis forward, keeping the weight in the heels. Continue to stretch arms and head back. Hold for 3 breaths.

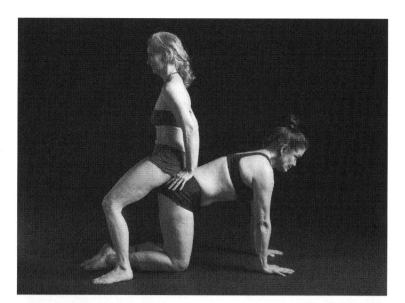

Massage Table

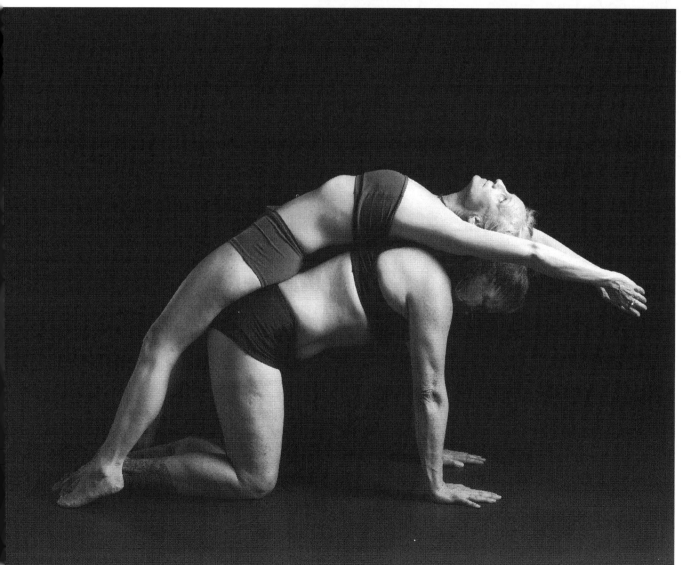

This partner posture combines the benefits of backward bending with the additional elements of allowing another being to hold and support you. You, in turn, get to hold and support them while they are completely vulnerable, putting their trust in you. Making the relationship reciprocal nourishes the development of strength and builds the ability to both give and receive support.

Partner 1 is on hands and knees. Make sure to line up hands directly under shoulders and knees under hips to form a strong base. Partner 2 gently reclines unto Partner 1's back, letting head rest on Partner 1's spine. Arms can hang down or extend over head to deepen the stretch. Partner 2's job is to relax and allow partner 1 to bear the weight. Remember, this is about developing more trust, hope and faith. Switch.

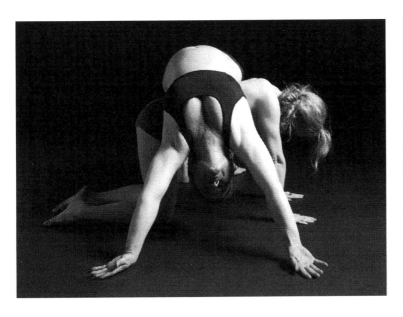

If Partner 2 has a flexible spine, this posture can be done crosswise.

Physical Benefits

PARTNER 1

- Tones arms and legs
- Tightens abdominal muscles
- Strengthens back

PARTNER 2

- Releases tension in shoulders and back
- Opens heart and throat chakras
- Allows relaxation in an open and vulnerable position

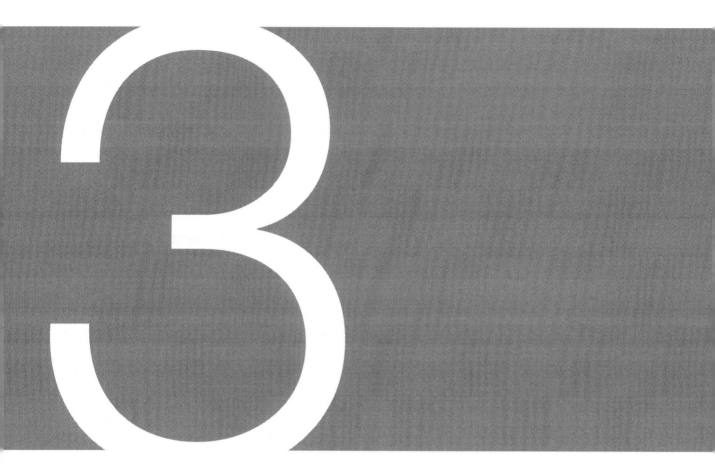

STEP THREE

Decision & Submission

- **Half Tortoise**
- **Standing Head to Knee**
- **Hanging Lift**

"Made a decision to turn our will and our lives over to the care of God as we understood Him."

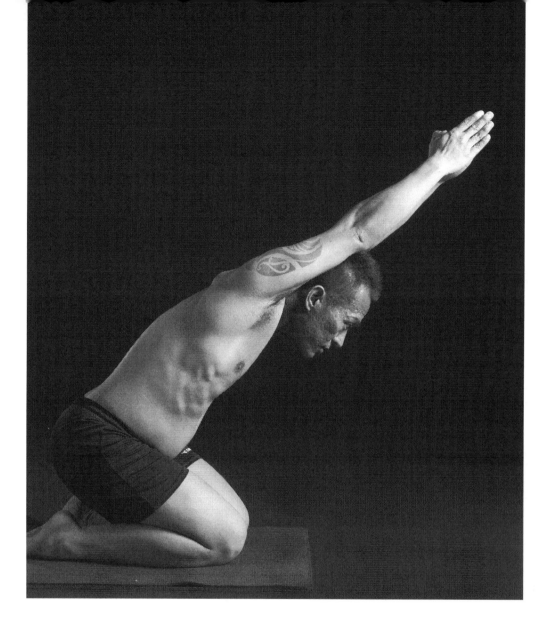

Half Tortoise *Ardha Kurmasana*

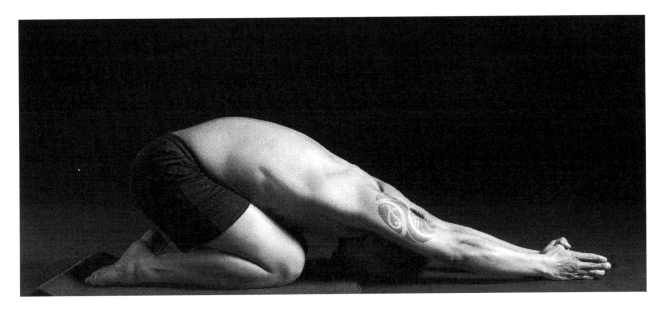

This posture is literally a bowing down. It is a position associated with submission and prayer in many cultures. Submission is a difficult idea to comprehend and come to terms with. Prayer does not come easily to everyone seeking recovery. In addition to the physiological benefits of this posture, it offers the opportunity to practice the act of submission. Bring the body and the mind will follow.

Sit, kneeling in vajrasana (hips on heels). Bring arms overhead, palms in prayer position, thumbs crossed. Inhale, extend up, chin away from the chest. Suck your stomach muscles in and bend forward, hinging at the hips. Come down, spine straight until forehead touches the floor. Keep extending arms overhead, pressing palms together and lifting wrists. Settle hips down unto heels. From belly button up stretching spine forward, from belly button down, stretching spine back. To come out, use abdominal muscles, bring spine upright, keeping hips on heels.

Physical Benefits

- Improves digestion
- Increases flexibility of hips and back
- Brings additional blood flow to brain

Standing Head to Knee *Dandayamana-Janushirasana*

There are four steps in this pose. Make sure to accomplish them in order. Do not move ahead until you have built a firm foundation. If you let your ego drive you to progress too fast, you only cheat yourself. You have to build a strong foundation, paying particular attention to the beginning, just like in recovery. It does no good to jump ahead if you haven't solidified your base. In yoga, jumping ahead can get you hurt. In recovery, it will get you loaded. In developing mental discipline, the specific task you chose to focus on does not matter. As Bikram says, "It is the trying itself that counts. The task just needs to be sufficiently challenging or daunting….and offer attractive enough rewards to make the effort worthwhile." In saying these words he could be talking about locking your knee or about working the steps as a path to recovery.

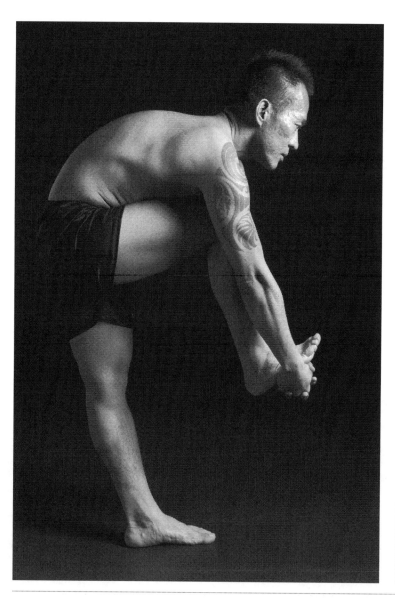

Physical Benefits

- Tightens abdominal and thigh muscles
- Increases flexibility entire back of leg
- Develops concentration and balance

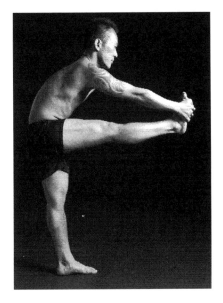 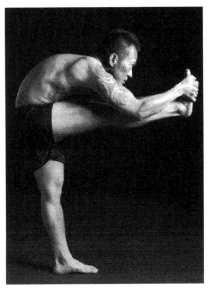 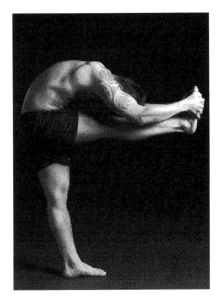

Stand with feet together. Transfer weight to your left leg. Lock out the left knee. Locking the knee is accomplished by contracting the muscles of the thigh. This includes the little muscles above the knee cap. Pick up the right foot. Hold it two inches below the toes. The foot should be directly under the knee with the thigh parallel to the floor so the leg forms a 90 degree angle. THE ONLY THING THAT MATTERS IN THIS POSTURE IS KEEPING THE STANDING KNEE LOCKED.

Try to hold for 30 seconds to begin with working up to one minute. Every time your knee bends, lock it out. The locked knee is a single minded, single point of focus. It is a mantra, a meditation. You make a decision to lock the standing knee and require the body to carry it out. It is mind over matter. Your brain is telling your body what to do. If you are unable to keep your knee locked for the full time holding the foot, back off and stand on your left leg with the right foot raised, thigh parallel to the floor. Stay here until you develop the strength to proceed. This requires the exercise of mental discipline. Do not let your ego push you too far. In addition to mental discipline, you get to work on patience. Patience, discipline and getting control of your ego, all by just locking your knee and keeping it locked!

Once you can lock the knee, the second step is to kick the right heel forward pulling toes back toward the face. Sucking in the stomach muscles really helps. You are kicking the right foot away from the body with the foot flexed. The goal is to get both knees locked. Once the kicking leg is locked, step three is to bend the elbows down alongside the calf muscles. Final expression is to lower the head and place the forehead on the knee. Come out of the posture opposite of the way you went in. Repeat on the other side.

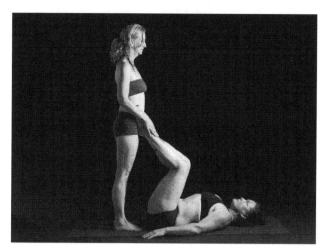
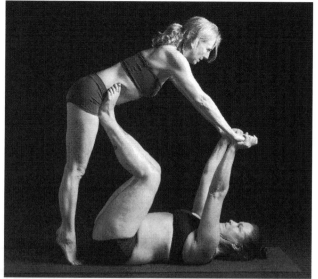
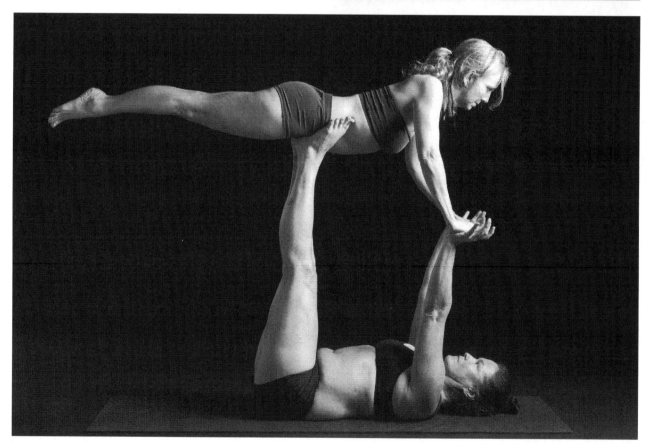

Hanging Lifts

The key to a successful lift is alignment. If the bones are properly stacked upon each other, physics does the work. ***Important:*** *Lifts are contraindicated for people with spinal or neck injuries, high blood pressure, a history of strokes, and women who are pregnant.*

Lifts are not for everyone. They can be risky. They are often tricky, especially in the beginning. Always practice in a clear, open space with a soft surface for landing. Be prepared to fall. Falling is part of the process. One of the hallmarks of practicing healthy relationships is recognizing failure is an essential part of the path to mastery. Lifts require courage, trust, good, clear communication, and belief in someone other than yourself. All excellent traits to practice in working recovery.

BASIC LIFT

Partner 1 lies on back, pressing lower back into the mat. Partner 1 bends knees and lifts feet off the floor. Partner 2 stands in front of Partner 1, placing hips on the lifted feet. Partner 2 then leans forward, releasing some of the body weight onto Partner 1's feet. Both partners extend arms toward each other and touch hands, palms flat. This is the foundation for the lift. Once the foundation is stable, Partner 2 takes small steps forward, continuing to lean weight into Partner 1's feet. Partner 1 allows knees to bend and thighs to move back toward the chest. Eventually, Partner 1's feet line up over hips.

When you have achieved this alignment, Partner 1 begins to straighten knees and lift Partner 2 off the ground. Once Partner 1 has legs comfortably straight, check to make sure feet are directly over hips. Arms are straight and lined up right over shoulders. Partner 2 presses down with hands and lifts head. Try to hold for 10 seconds. Breathe slowly and dismount carefully.

HANGING LIFT

Once you are comfortable with the basic lift, you can proceed to the hanging lift. Do the first bit, then release hands. Partner 2 hinges at the hips and allows body to hang, completely supported by Partner 1. Always reverse so both partners get to experience supporting and being supported.

Physical Benefits

PARTNER 1

- Strengthens thighs
- Stretches calves and hamstrings
- Develops concentration

PARTNER 2

- Releases tension neck and shoulders
- Reverses effects of gravity on spine
- Increases blood flow to head and face

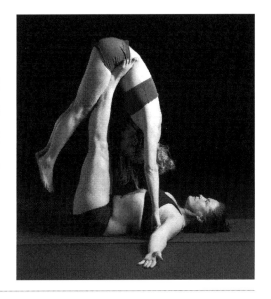

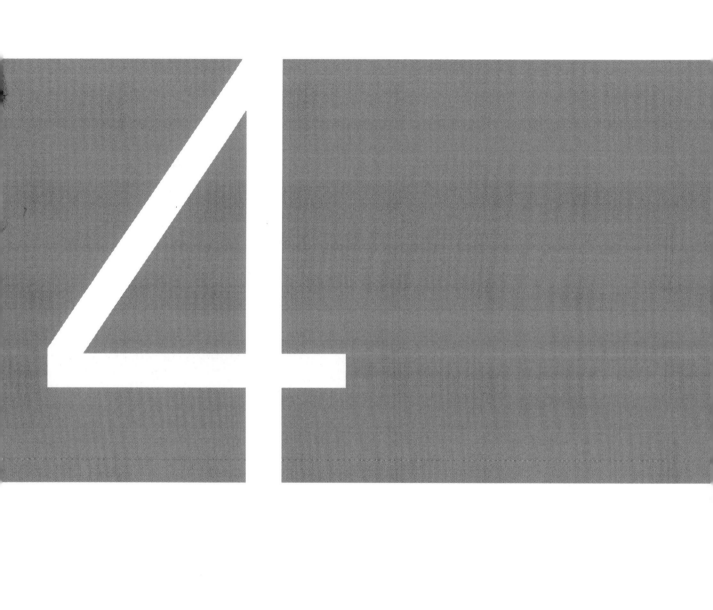

STEP FOUR

Courage & Self Awareness

- Warrior I
- Chair
- Breathe with Me

"Made a searching and fearless moral inventory of ourselves."

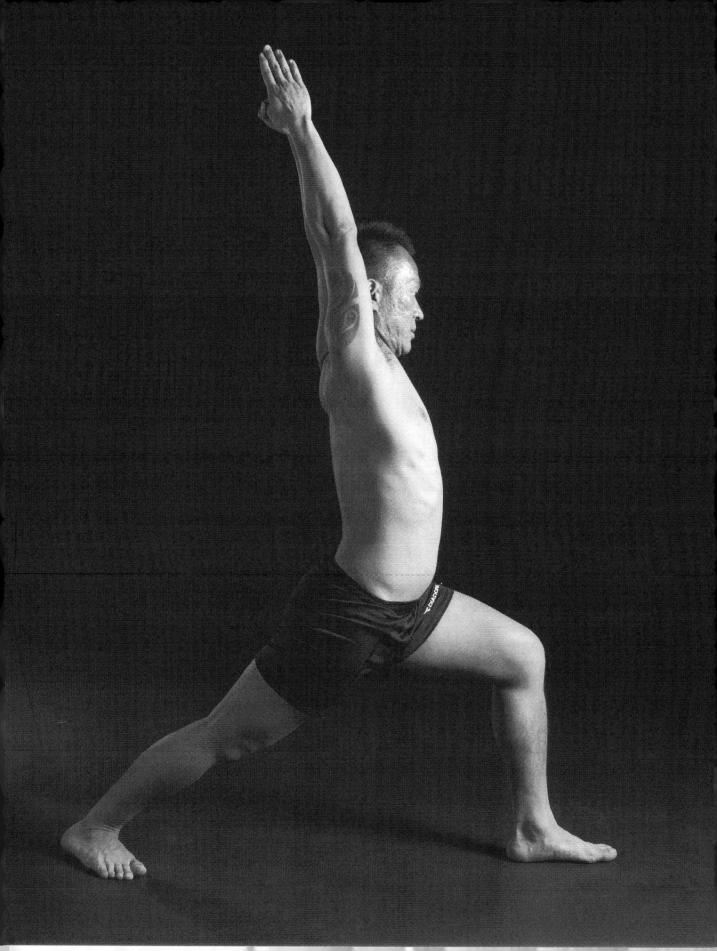

Warrior I *Virabhadrasana*

Imagine being a warrior, fighting for the triumph of good over evil, sobriety over addiction, serenity over insanity. Feel the energy of the posture as it strengthens the body and invigorates the mind. The chest lifts and opens allowing more room for the heart and lungs to expand.

Stand with feet together. Take a big step forward with the right foot. Right toes point forward. Left foot is at a 45 degree angle. Bend the right knee and drop the hips down until the thigh is at a 90 degree angle, parallel to the floor. Hips should point forward. Raise arms over head, palms together and flat, fingers touching. Drop shoulders and sink down into hips. Hold for four long slow deep breaths. Step together. Repeat with left leg forward.

Physical Benefits

- Stretches chest and lungs
- Opens hips and shoulders
- Strengthens thighs, calves and ankles

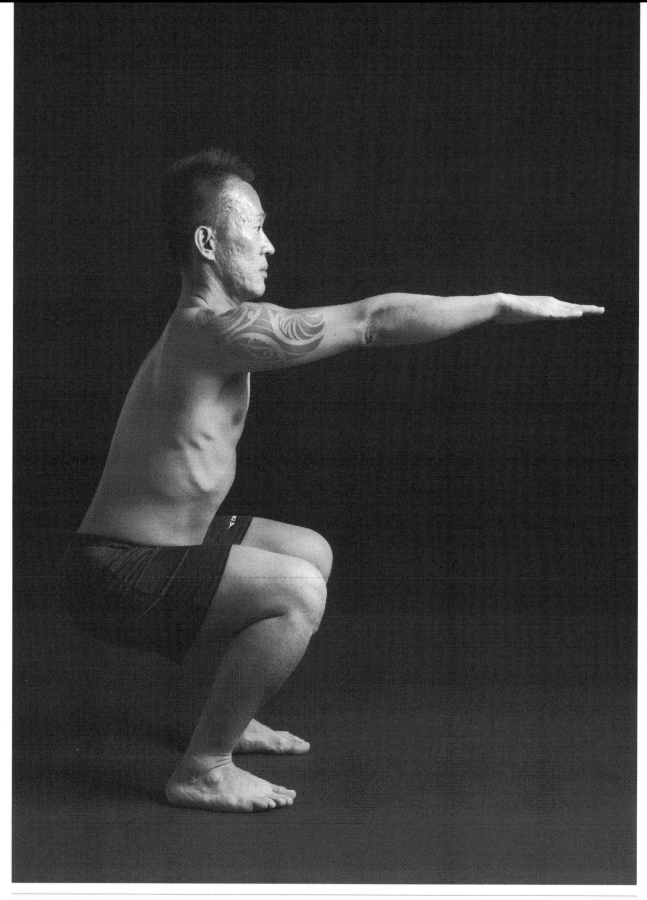

Physical Benefits

- Strengthens thighs, hips, calves and upper arms
- Increases flexibility in hip
- Brings more blood flow to ankles and knees

Chair *Utkatasana*

This posture develops power in the arms, legs and abdomen. It requires focused self-awareness to maintain the spacing and correct alignment. Then you work on developing determination and endurance as you build greater strength.

Stand with feet shoulder width apart. Extend the arms out in front, parallel to the floor. Contract all of the muscles in the arms, imagining energy shooting out of the finger tips. Press the shoulders down and back. Stick your butt out and sit down. Bend your knees until your thighs come down parallel to the floor. Keep knees over feet. Continue to bring shoulders back as fingers stretch forward. Hold for at least four breaths, longer as you get stronger.

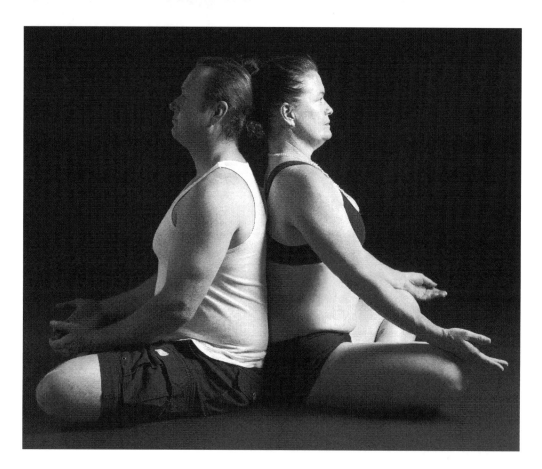

Breath with Me

Yoga is the marriage of the heart and lungs, mind and body, body and breath. Practicing yoga allows you to begin to develop an intimate relationship with your own body. In this exercise, we expand the sphere of intimacy to include another person. You get to explore the possibility of interpersonal intimacy within the privacy of your own breath. It provides a safe entre into difficult territory. Because you are back to back with your partner, eyes closed, you have the opportunity to explore your internal experience as you open yourself up to some one else. The amount you can learn about yourself in a vacuum is limited. It is through connection with others that more is revealed.

Breathe with Me is a powerful tool for developing self understanding. Connect your breath with your partner and watch the reactions in your mind and body. Use this information when you approach your searching and fearless moral inventory. It could shed light on many aspects of your fourth step. You are also laying the groundwork for moving on to step five where you share more than your breath with another human being.

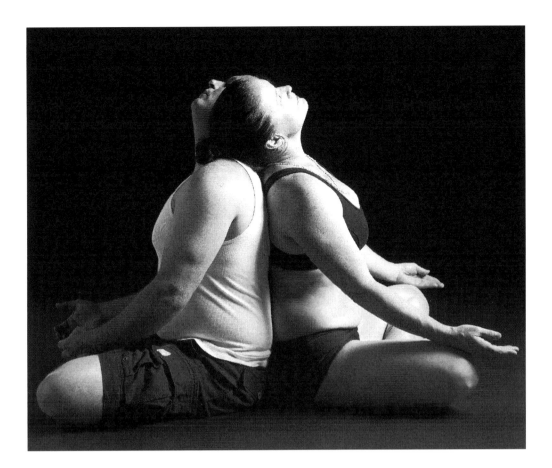

Sit comfortably, back to back. Make sure there is as much contact as possible from the base of the spine through the back of the head. Maximize contact without straining. Close your eyes and turn your attention to your breath. Follow each inhale as the lungs fill with air and expand. Stay with the exhale as air flows out, lungs deflate and chest relaxes. Try not to control the breath. Allow it flow naturally, in and out.

Do this for ten breaths, maintaining contact with partner's back throughout. On the eleventh breath, start to concentrate on your partner's breath. Expand the sphere of your awareness to include another person. Focus on your partner's lungs as they expand and contract. Feel the movement of their back against yours. In connecting this way you start to connect to that force which is breathing both of you.

In his poem, "The Third Body," Robert Bly talks about two people's breath creating a third entity. Bly states that when two people are breathing together they, "Feed someone we do not know…Someone we know of, whom we have never seen." I believe breathing together creates a connection with a higher power. This is the third body Bly is talking about. Khalil Gibran said this differently. He said, "It is in that vast man that we are vast." Either way, breathing together connects us to something greater than ourselves.

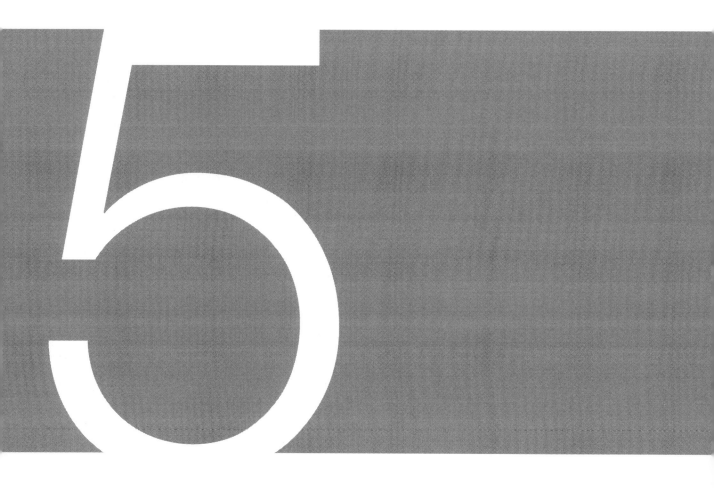

STEP FIVE

Honesty, Self Expression & Trust

- **Lion**
- **Standing Bow**
- **Backpack**

"Admitted to God, to ourselves, and to another human being the exact nature of your wrongs."

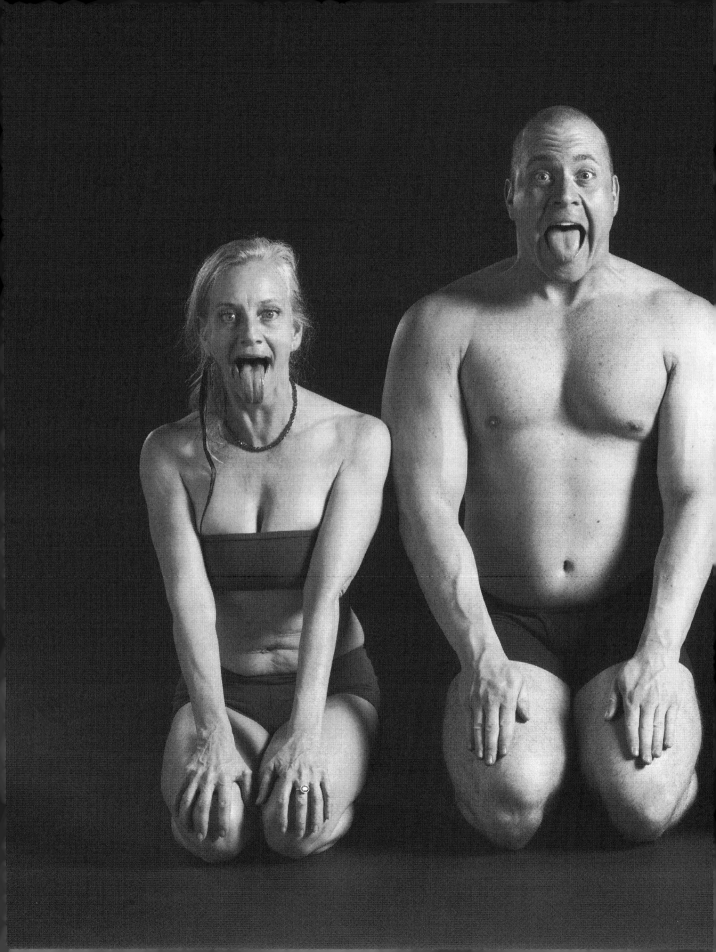

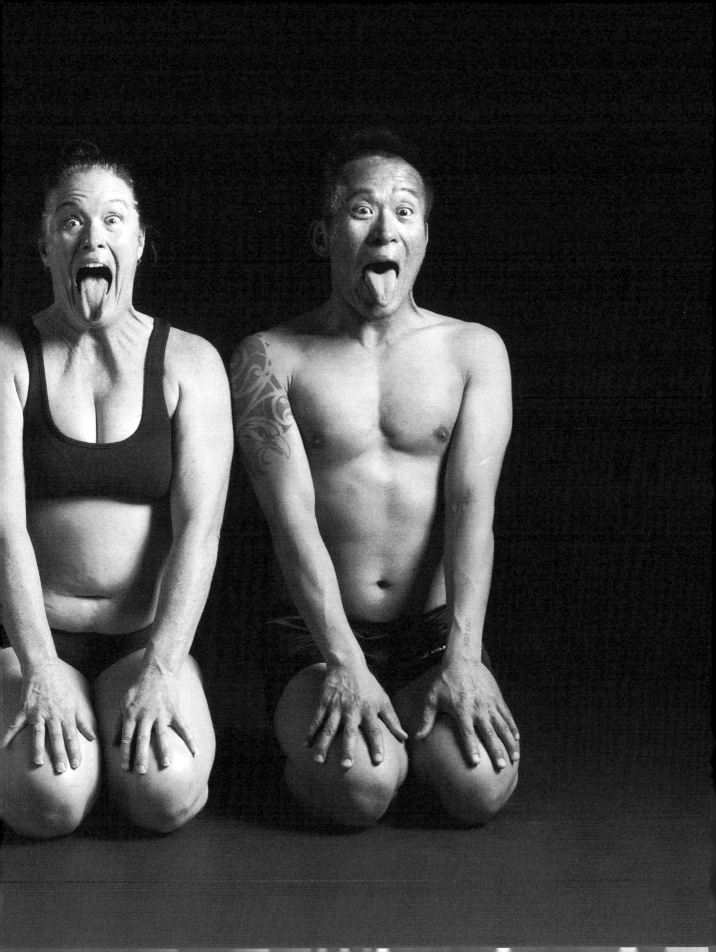

Lion *Simhasana*

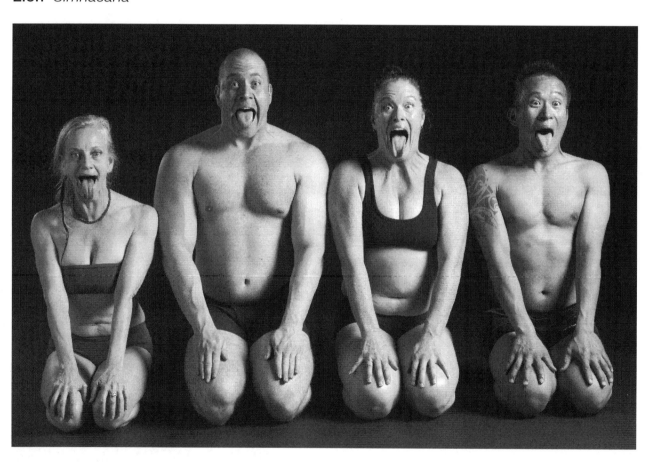

Physical Benefits

- Increases circulation to the face
- Relieves tension in jaw, neck and chest
- Stimulates optic nerve

Lion works with the TMJ, the place where your jaw hinges when you open your mouth. Many people store stress in this area, often without realizing it. Lion helps to release this tension. It is also really good for strengthening and releasing the throat chakra, helping people find their voice. Lion encourages self-expression. It is very simple. It can also be a lot of fun. The power of doing something that feels foolish should not be underestimated. There is a great deal of energy in stepping into that space. Some find it to be very liberating. Enjoy yourself.

Sit with hands on knees. Inhale deeply. As you exhale, open your mouth wide and stick your tongue out as for as it will go. Open eyes wide and roll them to back of head. Vocalization is optional, but the benefits increase when sound is included, so give it a try.

I encourage my students to either roar like a lion, or release whatever sound arises naturally, preferably with some strength and volume. Practice this three times, taking deep, full lung breaths in between.

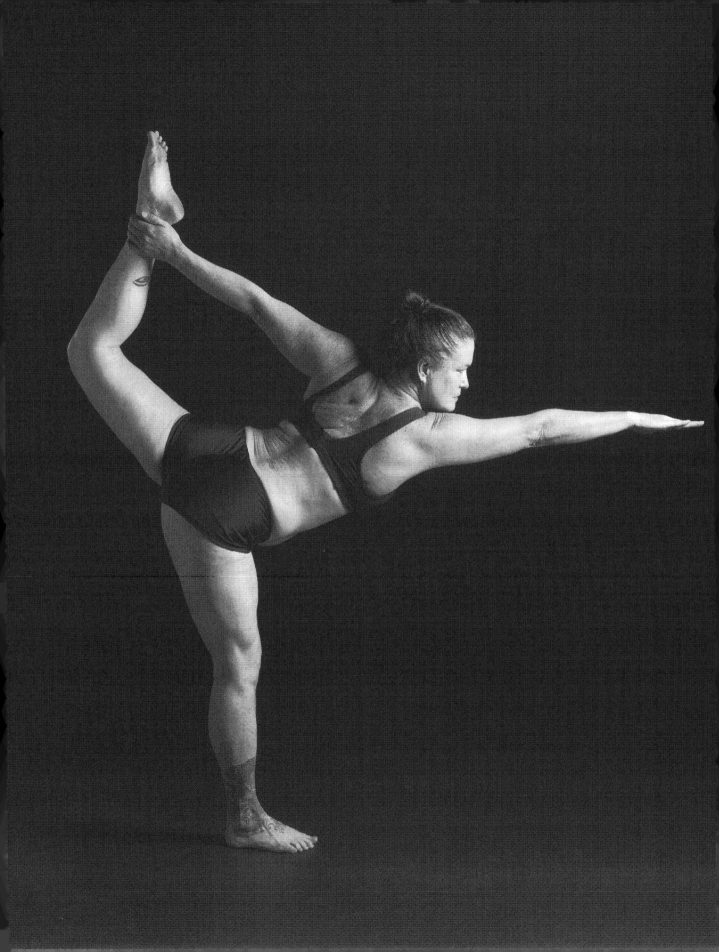

Standing Bow *Dandayamana-Dhanurasana*

Most people enjoy this posture and want to do it well. When you are in the posture, chest open, arms extended in opposite directions, it is the perfect embodiment of self expression. The gaze, the driste, is focused on the third eye point. All the energy is going forward.

Stand with feet together. Take your right elbow and place it at your waist, hand extended and palm up. Bring your hand back without flipping it over. Pick up your right foot, holding from the inside at the ankle. Bring your knees together to align your hips. Extend your left arm up to the ceiling, chin to the left shoulder. Begin kicking back and up. At the same time bring the chest and abdomen down. Keep arm up so fingers line up with third eye point (between the eyebrows). Focus the eyes on that point. Kick and reach and try to achieve balance. Remember balance is an unstable equilibrium. It is the opposing forces, working together, that allow one to feel stable and even.

Feel your arms being pulled apart in opposite directions. Notice what is happening inside your chest as the physical space expands. Come out gracefully and repeat on left side. Stand still and notice your internal environment. This posture shunts the volume of your blood flow from one side to the other. Stand still and breathe, allow everything to come back into equilibrium.

Physical Benefits

- Increases size and elasticity of lungs
- Firms and strengthens abdominal muscles, thighs, arms and buttocks
- Develops balance and concentration

Backpack

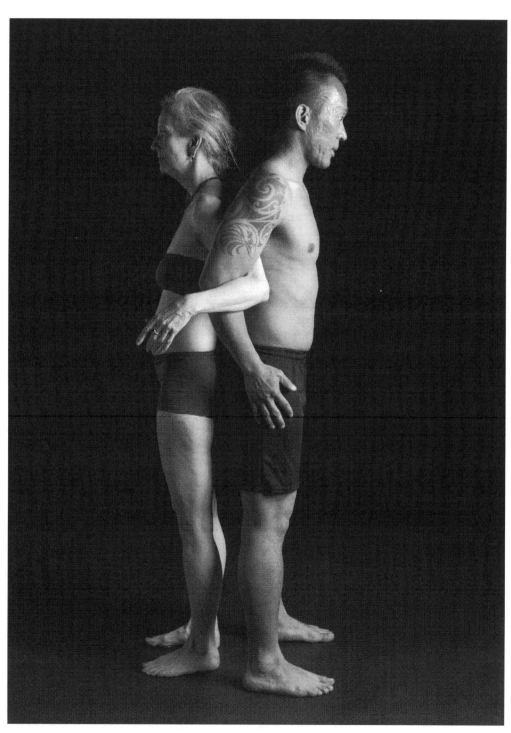

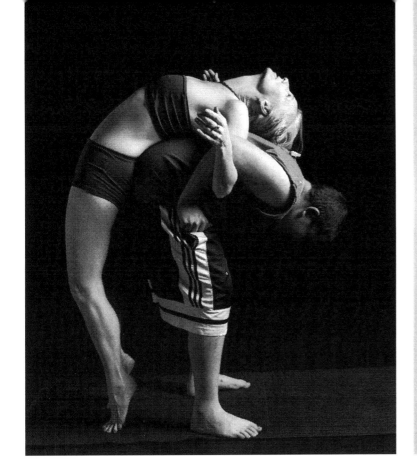

Physical Benefits

PARTNER 1

- Stretches and strengthens legs
- Increases blood flow to head
- Improves tone back and stomach muscles

PARTNER 2

- Opens chest
- Facilitates deep breathing
- Releases energy from spine

The benefits of this posture are similar to Massage Table, giving and receiving support. In addition, the strength of the standing position engages the legs, most people's most powerful muscles. This creates a stable supportive base for the second partner to relax and release into. Always have an agreed upon word for enough. "Stop," works really well.

Stand back to back with your partner. Link arms and extend spines against each other. Feet are shoulder width apart. Partner 1 will lift partner 2 first. Lifting is done more by leverage than strength. If you correctly position your buttocks on your partner's back, it will make the lift easier. Of course, this requires clear, direct communication and practice. Partner 1 takes a deep breath. On the exhale, bending forward, pulling in abdominal muscles to protect the lower spine. Partner 2 relaxes backward unto Partner 1, allowing themselves to be lifted.

STEP SIX

Cleansing & Willingness to Change

- Spinal Twist
- Shoulder Stand | Plough
- Assisted Hand Stand

"Were entirely ready to have God remove all these defects of character."

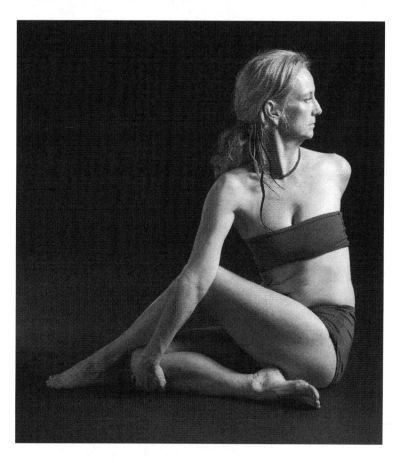

Spinal Twist *Ardha Matsendrasana*

This posture sounds complicated, but is totally worth the effort it takes to figure out where the elbows and knees connect. Twists are very detoxifying. This one wrings out your entire spine from bottom to top. Doing this regularly will help you cleanse and purify all the systems in your body.

Physical Benefits

- Improves flexibility of spine and hip joints
- Firms thighs, stomach and buttocks
- Increases circulation to spine and central nervous system

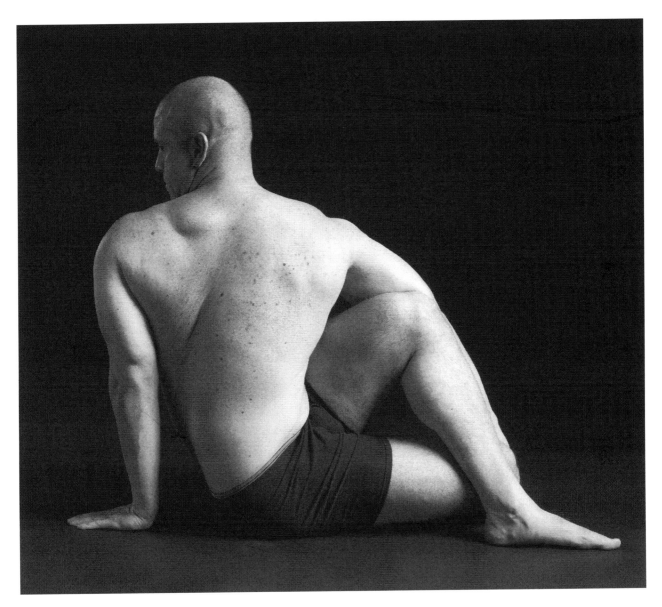

Sit on the floor with the left knee pointing forward and the left foot pointing behind you. Bring the right leg up and over, bending the right knee. Place the right heel at the outside of the left knee. Right hand goes behind you to straighten the spine. Left arm extends up, then left elbow is placed on the outside of the right knee and left hand on the left knee.

Take a deep breath and sit up straight. Begin twisting at the waist. Stay in the twist, straighten again and twist at the shoulders, opening the right shoulder behind you. Stay there and straighten up one more time. Twist your chin over your shoulder. Use your peripheral vision to look around as far as you can to the right. Release and repeat on the other side.

Cleansing and Willingness to Change

Shoulder Stand | Plough *Salamba Sarvangasana | Halasana*

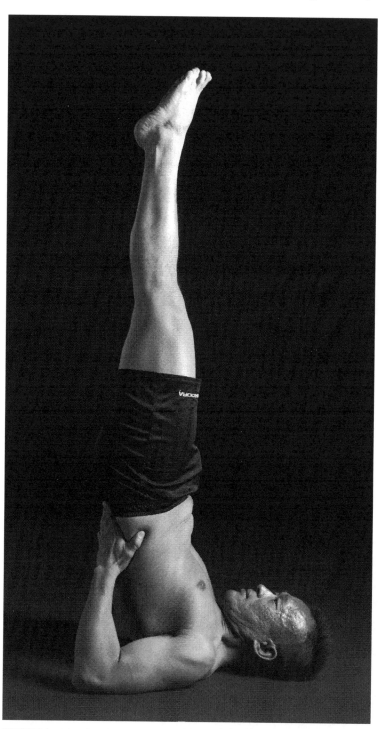

Inversions flip your energy, allow it to flow more freely and create new possibilities. If I'm interacting with someone and we feel stuck, I will often invert (stand on my head if the setting allows) to shift things around and get a different perspective. Shoulder stand is a less extreme inversion that should be accessible to most people. Also see Legs up the Wall pose in Flows at the back.

Physical Benefits

- Stimulates abdominal organs and thyroid gland
- Stretches shoulders and spine
- Reduces backache, headache and insomnia

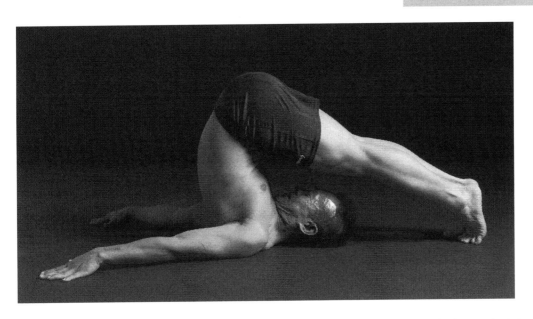

Lie on your back, legs together. Raise legs, rolling backward unto upper back and neck. Head is on the floor. Place hands on the lower back to support the spine. Chin is tucked into the chest. Relax and breathe, sinking down and stretching the cervical spine. Legs extend up to ceiling. If you want you can point toes and stretch legs up, increasing the bend at the neck.

To go into Plough, lower feet to floor, behind head. Arms can stay supporting the spine or extend away from feet along the floor. To come out, support your spine and roll down slowly, paying attention to the entire back as you roll down to the floor.

Cleansing and Willingness to Change

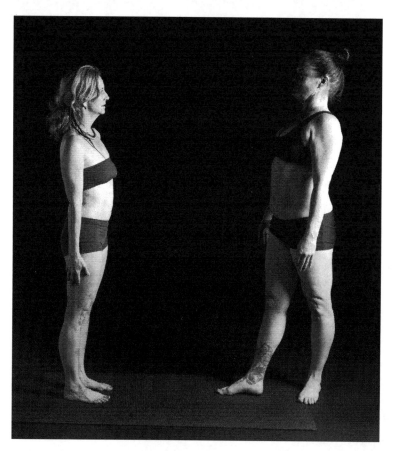

Many people never even consider doing a handstand. Or, they have not tried one since they were nine or ten. Either way, there is a great deal to be gained by accepting the adventure and taking the risk. Doing so with a partner—someone who is there to catch, support and steady you—can make it a much more appealing and also rewarding proposition. Doing the catching equals accepting responsibility. You are volunteering to show up for your partner and make sure they are safe while they, literally, take that leap of faith. Make sure to establish simple verbal cues such as, "Up, down, and stop."

Assisted Hand Stand

Stand facing one another, about three feet apart. Partner 1 has feet shoulder width apart and arms raised to catch Partner 2's legs. Partner 2 places palms on the floor about a foot from Partner 1's feet. Line up hands underneath the shoulders. Spread fingers apart, palms flat for maximum contact with the floor. Partner 2 bends knees slightly and prepares to kick up into Partner 1's hands.

To kick up, take a deep breath and push shoulders away from hands, engaging arms. On the exhale, bend one knee and straighten the other. Swing straight leg up and toward partner's hands. Straighten both legs and point toes to ceiling. Contract abdominal muscles and tighten buttocks. Continuously push away from the floor with arms as you stretch body and legs up.

Partner 1's job is to provide stability and support. Both partners concentrate on keeping spines straight. Hold for at least three breaths. Switch places and repeat.

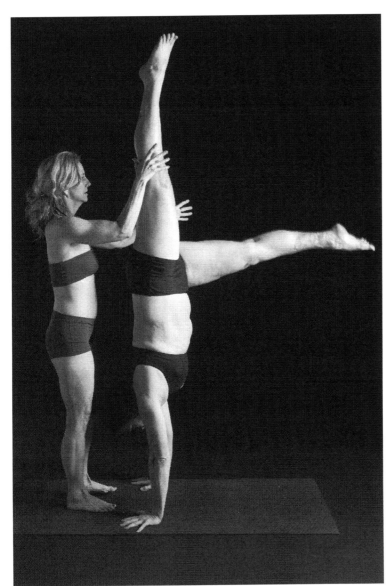
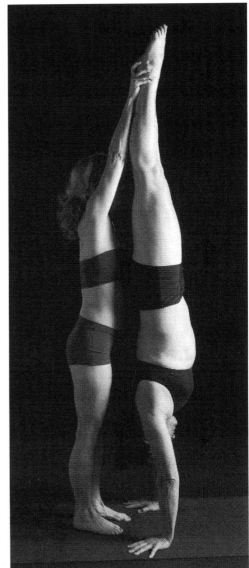

Physical Benefits

PARTNER 1

- Encourages upward flow of energy
- Increases awareness of posture
- Provides opportunity to accept responsibility

PARTNER 2

- Strengthens arms and shoulders
- Increases circulation to brain
- Stimulates pituitary gland

STEP SEVEN

Humility & Falling Short of the Mark

- **Downward Dog**
- **Camel**
- **Honoring**

"Humbly asked Him to remove our shortcomings."

Downward Dog *Adho Mukha Svanasana*

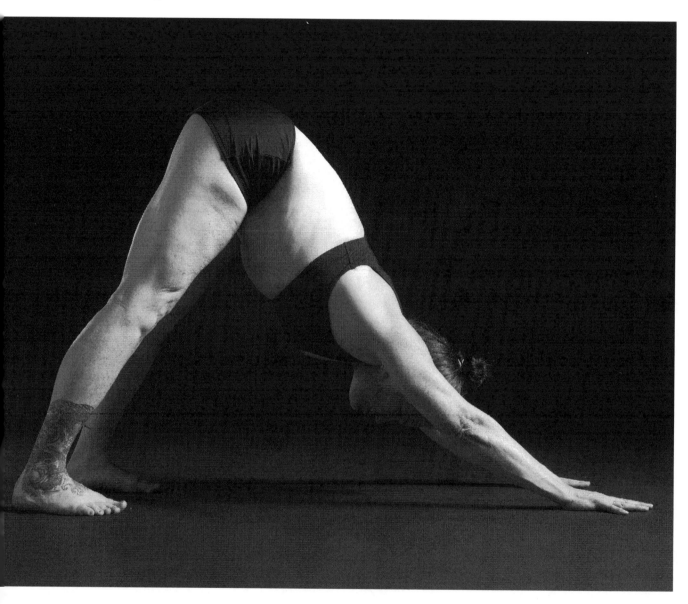

Physical Benefits

- Strengthens arms and legs
- Stretches shoulders, hamstrings and calves
- Calms brain and energizes body

Similar to Half-Tortoise, Downward Dog puts the student in a humbling position. It is also an inversion, bringing the head below the heart. Metaphorically, you are bowing the head (thinking) to the heart (feeling). Physiologically you are bringing blood with oxygen and nutrients to the brain. Energetically it serves the purpose of all inversions, flipping the flow of energy, releasing restrictions and creating greater possibilities.

Come onto the mat on hands and knees. Place knees directly below hips and hands slightly forward of elbows. Spread palms against the floor. Exhale and lift knees. At first knees are bent and heels can come off mat, arms are straight.

Press heels down toward floor as you push back and up, lengthening shoulders away from hands. Stretch tailbone toward ceiling and a little bit forward. Hold position and breathe, continuing to push down through the arms and lift the hips.

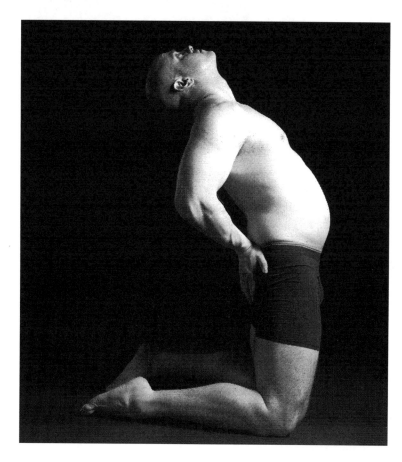

Camel *Ustrasana*

This posture is a huge heart opener. In a *Yoga Journal* article, Camel is referred to as, "Blasting the heart chakra open." It is also very difficult. Most students, at least in the beginning must accept that they cannot do the posture properly, let alone to its fullest expression. However, if you practice with diligence, patience, and humility, it will improve.

Because of the intensity of the backward bend, and the opening through the hips and pelvis, Camel brings up enormous emotional content. This can manifest as dizziness, nausea, anger, fear, sadness, or unexpected laughter. I encourage my students not to attach meaning to what arises during and after camel. Rather I suggest they acknowledge the sensations. It works best to stay with the feelings while in the pose and allow them to dissipate with the exhale in savasana.

Being humble requires vulnerability. Admitting to shortcomings is the opposite of being defensive. In Camel, the student is completely vulnerable. They are literally blindly baring their chest. Vulnerability is terrifying, difficult and essential for recovery. One of the definitions is, "Being open to attack." Being able to practice, to embody this openness in a safe arena, allows people to begin to exercise the "muscles" necessary to work the seventh step.

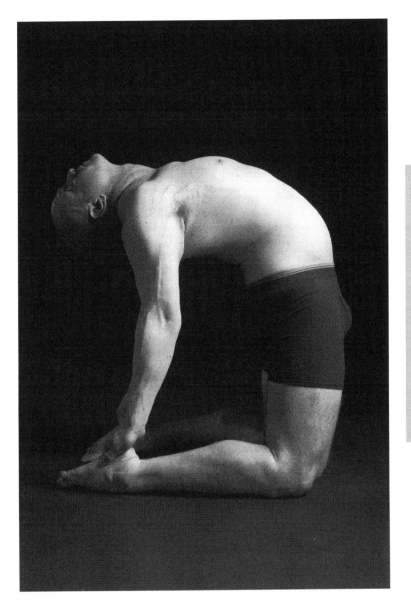

Physical Benefits

- Stretches abdominal organs
- Stretches throat, thyroid and parathyroid glands
- Increases flexibility and blood flow to the spine

Stand on knees, keeping feet and knees six inches apart. Place the hands on the lower back, with thumbs on the outside. This is to support the spine as you initiate the backward bend. Drop your head back as far as it goes. At the same time, push pelvis forward, contracting buttocks. Keep this forward motion constant throughout posture. Pause in the first position. If you can see the wall behind you, reach back and grab your heels one at a time. Grip the heels tightly.

There are two motions in the posture. You push the hips forward and lift the chest up. Close the mouth, intensifying stretch across the front of the neck. Keep pushing forward and lifting up. To come out, SUPPORT THE BACK WITH THE HANDS. This is very important. You have just done a very deep back bend and want to make sure to support the spine as you roll up slowly.

Honoring

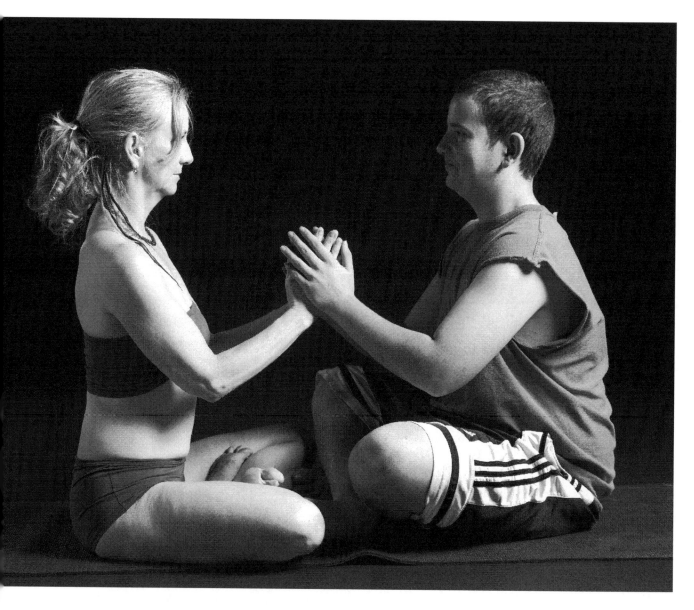

Honoring is an exercise in seeing and being seen. You sit before your partner, allowing them to see view you just as you are in that moment, in that place. In turn, you calmly and openly gaze at your partner. To allow another person to completely occupy your attention is an act of humility. Allowing yourself to be seen, just as you are, requires controlling your ego.

Sit in lotus or with legs crossed, knees touching. Partner 1 brings hands forward, palms together away from chest. Partner 2 places hands outside Partner1's, palms to the inside. Soften the gaze by releasing the little muscles around the eyeballs. Concentrate on seeing your partner as a whole being, in their entirety. Allow yourself to be viewed in the same way, just as you are. Try to give and receive attention equally without judgment. Hold for ten breathes and reverse hand placement. At the end, bring hands to the chest in namaskar and bow the head to the hands.

STEP EIGHT

Accountability & Changing Behavior

- Rabbit
- Tiger
- Double Tree / Lean on Me

"Made a list of all persons we had harmed and became willing to make amends to them all."

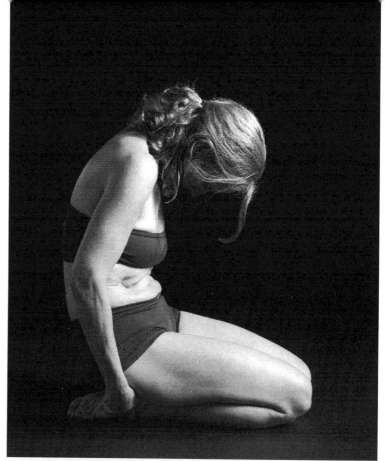

Rabbit *Sasangasana*

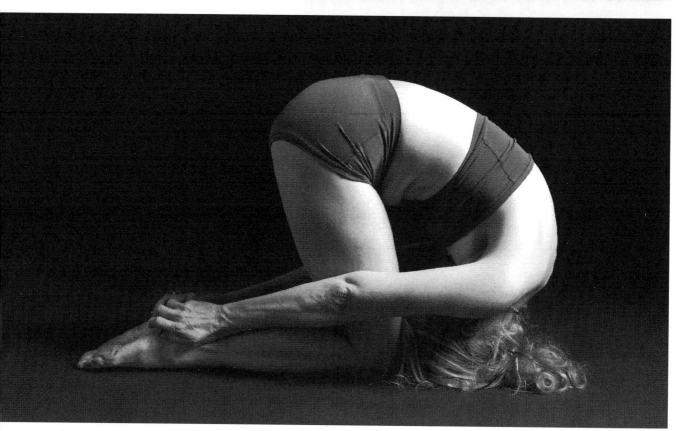

Physical Benefits

- Increased mobility of the spine
- Creates space between the vertebra, allowing discs to fall back to their natural alignment
- Compresses thyroid and parathyroid, regulates metabolism

In Rabbit you are rolling into yourself. You have no choice but to look at you. Even if you close your eyes you are still stuck, rolled up in a ball with yourself. To stay there, relax and breathe, allowing the integration of the self with the mind, the body with the breath.

Rabbit is a great diagnostic tool. With the spine rounded forward to its maximum ability it is possible for the trained observer to pinpoint where there are areas of constriction and decreased mobility. It is impossible to hide the truth about the spine in this position. This truth can then be mirrored back and real change becomes possible.

Kneel on the mat, hips on heels. Reach behind you and grab your heels. Use your whole palm to grip your heels, with the thumbs on the outside. Drop your head and round spine, contracting abdominal muscles. Tuck your chin into your chest, stretching the cervical spine.

Slowly round down until your head touches the floor in front of your knees. Ideally your forehead should touch the knees, but do not move your head once it is on the floor. Lift hips up to the ceiling, pulling on heels to take most of the weight in the arms, putting less pressure onto the top of the head. Look up at your belly button and suck stomach in, continuing to pull chin to chest. Breathe as normally as possible, keeping the stomach muscles contracted. Hold for at least a few long slow breaths. Coming out, roll up one vertebra at a time. Concentrate on your spine as you come up. Head comes up last.

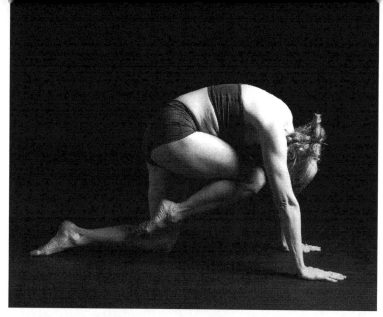

Tiger *Vyaghrasana*

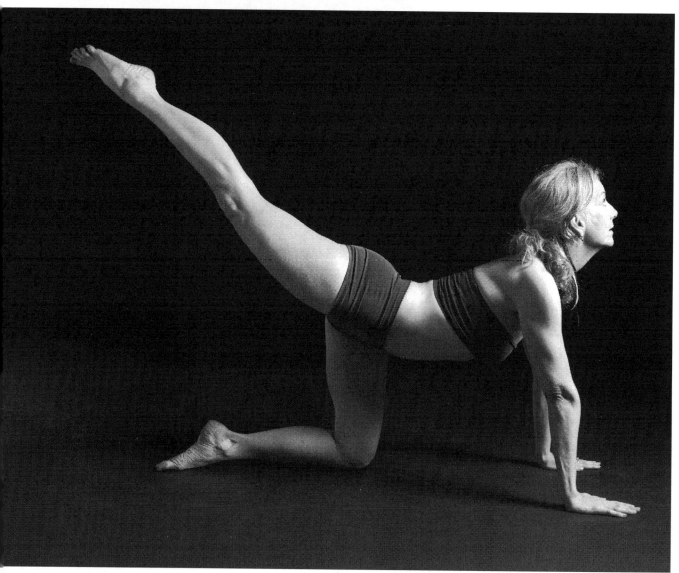

Step Eight

Having done some honest self examination, it is time to spring into action. In this pose, you are going from being a house cat to embodying the energy, the ferocity and the agility of a tiger.

Come to the mat on your hands and knees. Align knees below hips and hands under shoulders. Hands are palm down, fingers together and pointing forward. Arch your back and go into cat pose, pulling one leg in to chest, inhaling deeply.

As you exhale, extend bent leg back and up, pointing the toe and locking the knee. Hold this position for one breath. Do this gently, but with some energy. Repeat 3 times and then do on the other side.

Physical Benefits

- Tones spinal nerves
- Promotes digestion
- Stretches and revitalizes muscles in legs and buttocks

Double Tree / Lean on Me

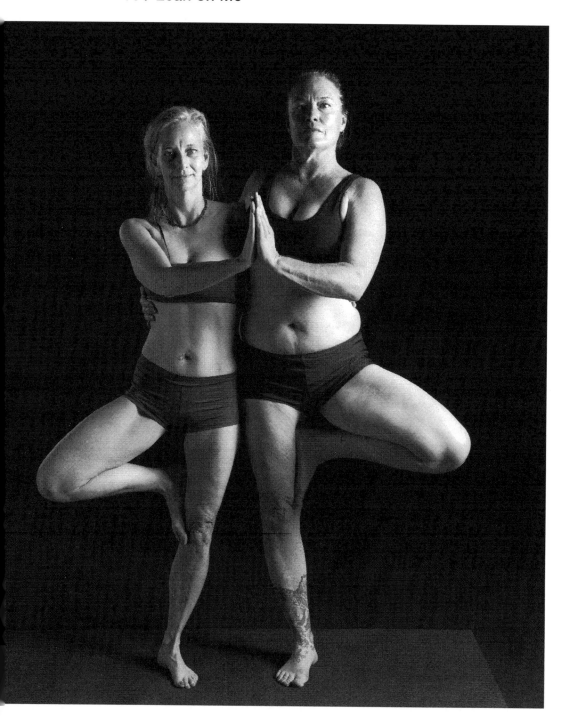

To do this posture, you have to lean on your partner, relying on them to help keep you balanced and standing up. It is impossible to accomplish Double Tree with individual effort. Relying on someone else did not come naturally or easily for me. I was unable to do so until I realized I could not stay sober without taking that risk. In recovery we have to learn to lean on each other. As with all partner postures, Double Tree offers the opportunity to practice this skill in a safe way with limited responsibilities and clear boundaries.

Stand side by side with hips touching. Experiment with spacing of the feet. Proper spacing will be determined by the height and weight differential of the partners. Start at approximately 10 inches and see what works best. Wrap inside arms around your partner's waist. Lift the outside leg and place foot on inside of standing leg. Bring outside hand to center, forming a 2-person namaskar. Balance and breathe.

Physical Benefits

- Increases flexibility of hips, knees and ankles
- Improves posture
- Increases concentration and balance

STEP NINE

Responsibility & Taking Action

- **Balancing Stick**
- **Pigeon**
- **Standing Twist**

"Made direct amends to such people wherever possible, except when to do so would injure them or others."

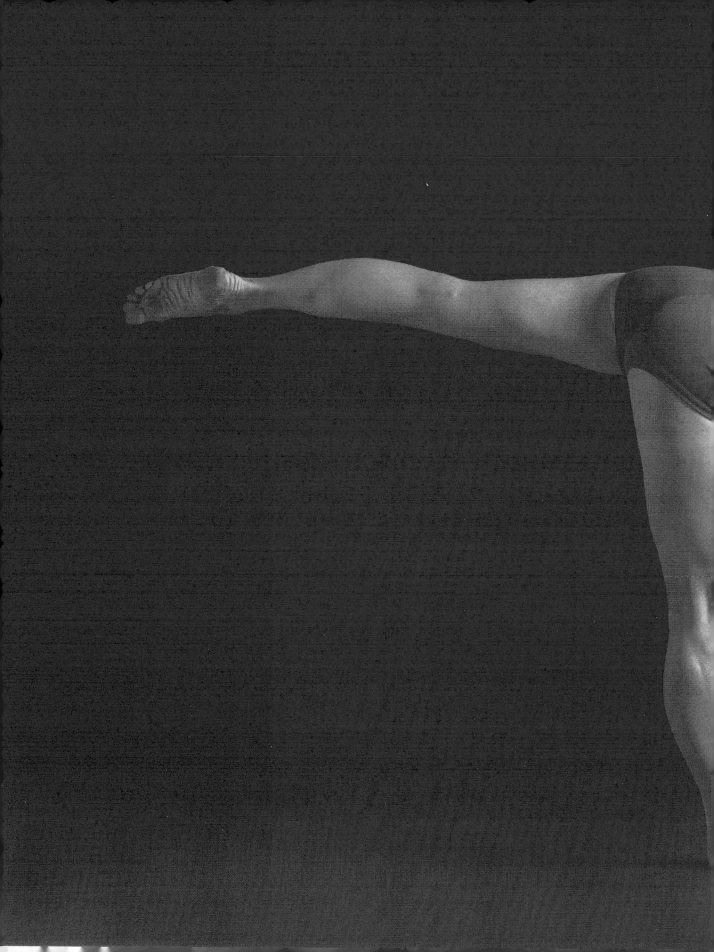

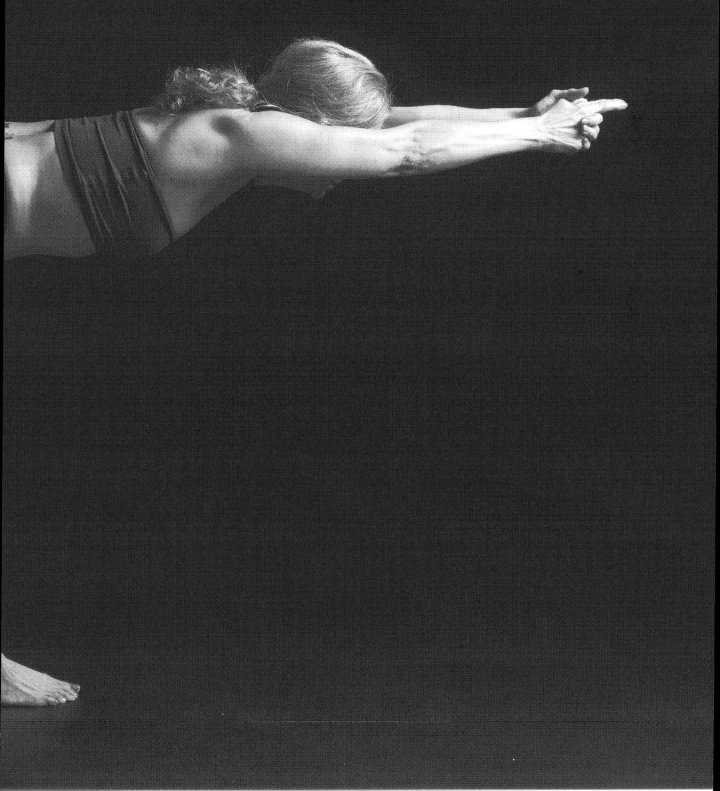

Balancing Stick Tulandasana

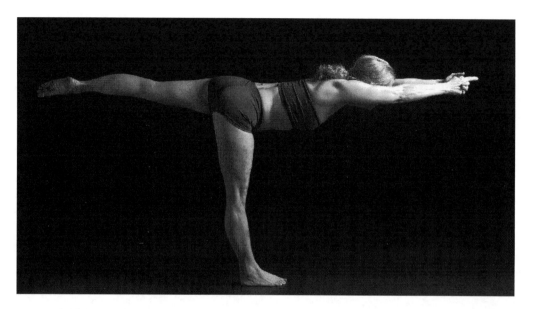

This posture greatly increases respiratory rate and heart rate. After 10 seconds in the posture, your heart is pounding and you may be gasping for air. By standing still, closing the mouth and breathing through the nose, you are accomplishing an amazing number of things. By greatly increasing the heart rate, you are artificially inducing physiological stress. The stress response is mediated by the sympathetic nervous system. Breathing through the nose and slowing the respiratory rate, you trigger a different neurological response, engaging the parasympathetic nervous pathway. Sympathetic is fight or flight. Parasympathetic sends the opposite signal to your system. It lets you know that everything is going to be alright, that nothing bad is happening. Practicing balancing stick, you can reprogram your stress response. You are teaching your body to relax on command. The command is given by taking long slow, even breathes in through the nose and out through the nose. You link the respiratory rate with the heart rate and slow everything down. Calming your body then serves to calm your mind.

Stand with feet together, arms over head fingers interlocked. Extend index fingers and press the palms together. Take a big step forward onto right foot. Point left toes, lifting left foot off ground, locking left knee. Inhale as you stretch up. Lock the right leg also and pivot forward from the hip, using the exhale to bring your body down and forward. You want to get everything perpendicular to the floor. Squeeze the head with the arms. Lift your legs and extend it behind you, keeping your toes pointed. From the waist up, you are stretching forward and from the waist back you are stretching back. Hold for ten seconds. Step back together and repeat with left leg forward. Complete one cycle and stand still, breathing through your nose.

Physical Benefits

- Firms hips, buttocks and upper thighs
- Strengthens the heart muscles
- Improves flexibility and strength in shoulders and upper arms

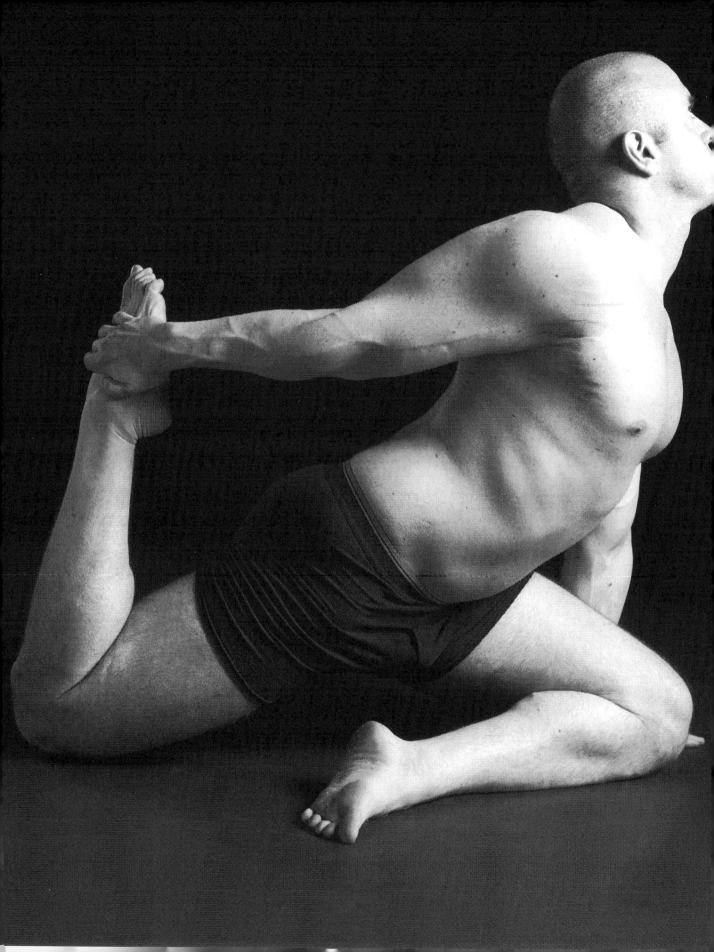

Physical Benefits

- Opens hips
- Stretches groin, psoas muscles and glutes
- Helps with urinary tract issues

Pigeon *Eka Pada Kapotasana*

Everyone who decides to work the steps has experienced trauma. For some it is from the effects of the addiction. Many have come from families where traumatic events took place. My own story includes a very difficult childhood, having surgery without being anesthetized, and the sudden death of my husband. Some of this happened before I started drinking, some after I got sober. The nasal deep breathing discussed in Balancing Stick is very helpful for trauma. So is working into some of the emotional issues.

Everything that happens is stored in the body. The hips and pelvis hold a great deal of emotional information. By physically loosening the joints and connective tissue that surround this area, you can begin to access and release emotional constrictions and scars. Be prepared for this. Move slowly and mindfully into your hips. Use your breath to calm your mind and heart. Try not to attach meaning to sensations as they arise. The beauty of yoga is you can work through emotional blockage and release them without having to label them or try to understand. Open your hips and your mind (and heart) will follow.

Sit, kneeling in vajrasana. Bring one leg in front of the other, bending the knee and sliding it forward. Make sure you are not sitting on the front foot. Extend the other leg behind you. Arms are alongside your body, palms flat on the floor. Support your body weight on your hands, controlling the intensity of the stretch through the hips. Use your breath by holding steady on the inhale and relaxing the pelvis toward the floor on the exhale. You can bend the back leg at the knee and grab your foot with same side hand to deepen the stretch and also work the front of your thigh.

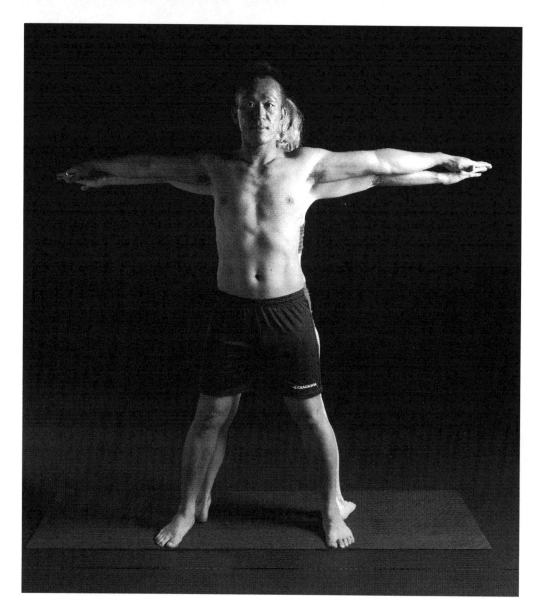

Standing Twist

Standing twist is a powerful partner posture that take a little practice and finesse to accomplish. It is dynamic. You are twisting the waist and opening across your chest. The primary point of contact is at the hip. All of these areas contain lots of emotional content. You get to access these parts of your body while synchronizing the movement and intention with another person. In addition to being enjoyable, it can also be a moving experience.

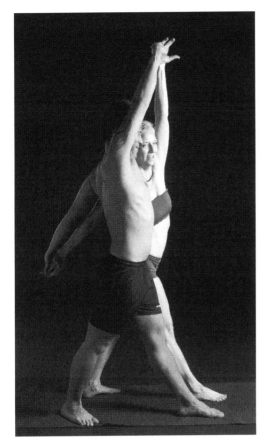 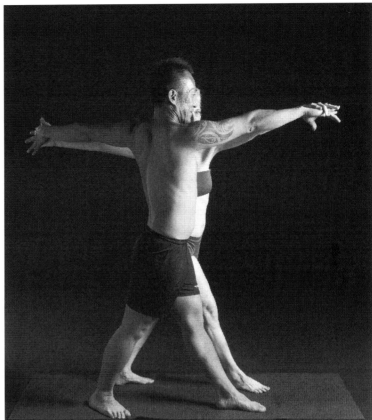

Stand back to back with your partner. Open feet about forty eight inches apart. Stretch your arms out to the side and hold hands. Both partners look in the same direction (one to the left, one to the right). Partner 1 turns left foot to the left. Partner 2 turns right foot to the right. Both partners drop inside arm and raise outside arm overhead. Keep hands in contact. Outside hips touch. Lower upper hand and raise lower hand. Upper bodies twist to the inside. Face one another. Breathe and smile. Open your heart to your partner. Look into each other's eye. Notice any feeling or sensations that arise, trying not to attach significance or meaning. Hold for several breaths. Repeat in opposite direction.

Physical Benefits

- Relieves tension in the chest, neck and shoulders
- Massages abdominal organs and stimulates kidneys
- Wrings toxins out of all systems

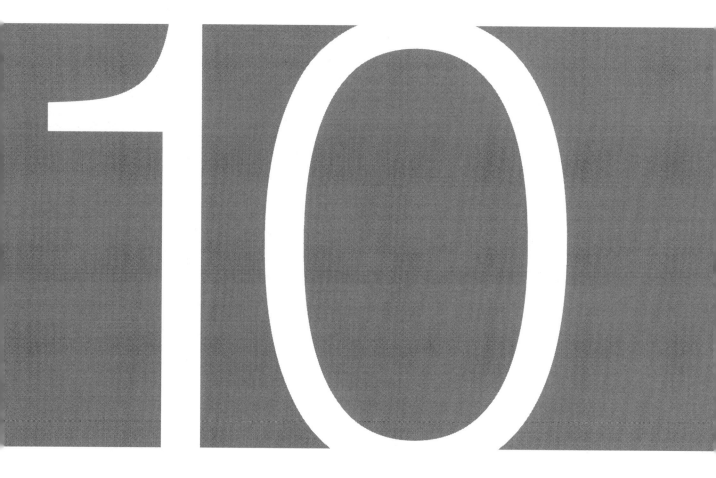

STEP TEN

Self Assessment

- Tree
- Eagle
- Double Triangle

"Continued to take personal inventory and when we were wrong, promptly admitted it."

Tree *Vriksasana*

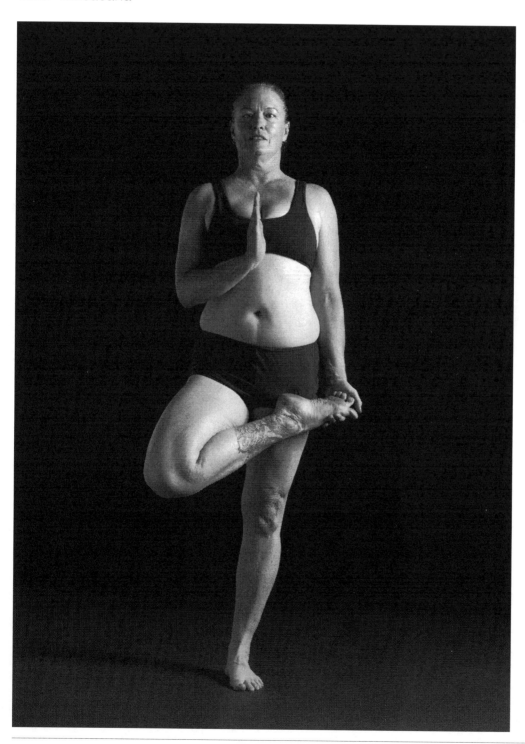

Step Ten

In addition to opening the hips knees and ankles, Tree is an exercise in self awareness. It can be very helpful to practice Tree in front of a mirror until you develop your internal sense of what level and balanced feels like.

Stand with feet together. Stand up tall as if there were a string attached to the top of your head, pulling you up to the ceiling. Transfer weight to left foot, rooting the foot firmly into the floor. Bring right foot up. There are many variations. You can bring it all the way up so the sole of the foot faces the ceiling and the heel is in the groin. Or you can place the sole of the right foot against the inner left thigh, gradually bringing the right foot higher up the standing leg. Pay close attention to your right knee, pressing it down and back, but not straining or going to the point of pain. Bring hands together in namaskar.

Scan through your body. You want to be balanced as if standing on both legs. Hips should be level, shoulders, eyebrows, ears, everything level. Stand up tall and think like a tree. Put down roots, feel the strength in your trunk and still the movements of your limbs.

Physical Benefits

- Opens hips, knees and ankles
- Improves posture
- Lengthens spine

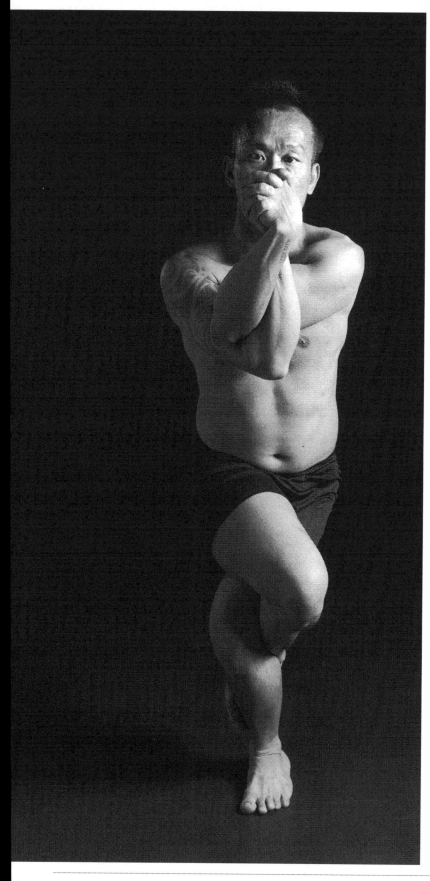

Eagle *Garasana*

Physical Benefits

- Opens all major joints in body
- Stretches upper back and shoulders
- Improves balance and concentration

Eagle is a great diagnostic posture. It works to open up all of the major joints in your body. By setting the goal of lining your arms and legs up in the middle of your body, you are able to see where you are out of alignment. Making sincere effort to shift and open joints that are constricted allows you to practice putting self-awareness into action. This is another posture that is helpful to practice in front of the mirror.

Stand with your feet together, arms over head. Bring your right arm under your left arm crossing at the elbow and again at the wrist. Wrap your wrists around each other, bringing palms together and thumbs toward the nose. Pull your elbows down and feel the stretch across your back. Suck your stomach in and bend your knees. Transfer weight to your left leg. Pick up your right foot and wrap your right leg around your left, crossing at the upper thighs.

The goal is to get the right toes tucked behind the left calf. If this is impossible, point the right toes down toward the floor. You want your ankles, knees, elbows and hands lined up right down the middle of your body. Make tiny movements toward the midline. Breathe deeply. An alternate version is to raise the arms up, keeping them crossed. This shifts the stretch to your upper arms and shoulders. Repeat with left arm under right, left leg over right. Notice if you're really different on one side or the other.

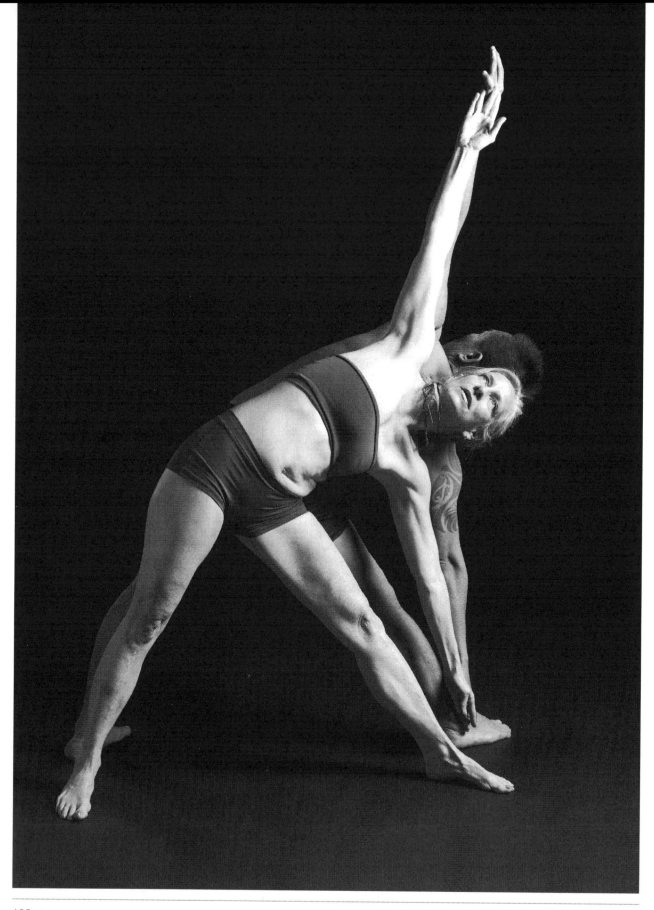

Double Triangle

Triangle is a master posture. It engages every fiber of your being. To engage deeply, while simultaneously leaning on and supporting your partner is an intense exercise in yoga and intimacy. Partners are mirroring each other's actions. This requires a high degree of self awareness as well as tuning in to the other person.

Stand back to back. Legs three to four feet apart. Partner 1 presses right hip to the right, Partner 2 presses left hip to the left. Both partners keep contact at the lower back and outside hip. Partner1 leans to the right, extending right arm down to the right foot, right leg straight. Partner 2 does the same to the left. Both extend other arm up to the sky, touching at the forearm or hand. Look up.

Feel the length of your back against your partner and breathe deeply. Come up slowly and repeat to the other side. You will have to experiment with your balance and the amount of weight you lean into each other. Your personal alignment is important to maintain the integrity of the whole posture.

Physical Benefits

- Tones spinal nerves
- Stimulates kidneys
- Improves blood flow to adrenal glands

STEP ELEVEN

Conscious Contact

- Savasana
- Lotus
- Double Savasana
- Double Lotus

"Sought through prayer and meditation to improve our conscious contact with God."

All yoga postures were created so practitioners could strengthen their bodies in order to sit longer in meditation. The asana serves the breath and the breath calms the mind. The mind is then stilled enough to turn more powerfully to meditation. Yoga is moving into stillness. As an introduction to meditation in stillness, one of the things I talk about in class is creating space. This space is a separation between thoughts and impulses. To practice we begin by creating a pause between having an idea and acting upon it. It is in this space that change becomes possible. By creating space one is able to consider alternative options. This process can be scary. T.S Elliot talks about its power in his poem, *The Hallow Men*.

> *A moment with the Beloved and the River changes its course.*
>
> Ram Dass

> *Between the concept*
> *And the action*
> *Between the emotion*
> *And the response*
> *Falls the shadow.*
>
> *Between the desire*
> *And the spasm*
> *Between the potency*
> *And the existence*
> *Falls the shadow*
>
> T.S. Elliot

Both Ram Dass and T.S Elliot understood the potency of this space. It creates room for the Divine to enter. It is also terrifying. In my own journey I have had to come to terms with the Shadow.

Coming to terms meant integrating those parts of my experience that caused me pain and of which I felt ashamed. I had to accept that shadow and joy were two sides of the same coin.

Finally, the direction within out shadow. This is the place I do not want my brothers and sisters to see, for I do not want to own it. Yet, my shadow holds me, so I invite my shadow to be seen. I do this so that I may accept the whole self that I am. My shadow holds so much of my gold. Shadow, know that you are safe here and will not be dishonored. Acceptance is the key to my spiritual growth. Thank you Shadow for once protecting me. Thank you for the purpose that you served. I bless my shadow by owning sharing and forgiving.

I wish you sweetness, honey in the heart, no evil, soberness, clarity and fulfillment.

Mayan Prayer

If I don't do ZEN meditation
to wipe out crazy thoughts
Then I must pace around drunkenly
spouting crazy songs.

Po Chu I, Chinese Poet,
12 hundred years ago

Savasana

I've had my addiction described as an impulse disorder. This makes tremendous sense to me. I began noticing all the places in my life where I acted on impulse without thinking things through. I understood the behavior, but did not know how to change. Practicing in savasana gave me a place to start. I began to get slivers of moment on the mat where I was able to create separation. Then I began to be able to inhabit the space I created. I became a witness. From this space I was able to evaluate the proposed action and consider the consequences. I learned to respond rather than react. This was totally new behavior for me.

In AA they tell you to Stop and Think. This sounds simple, but I needed a framework within which to establish this practice. Practicing savasana created an opening for me. The initial opening was tiny and progress was slow. This mirrors my beginning in recovery. I had the smallest inkling of a desire to change. In that tiny space, grace stepped in and I got sober.

Physical Benefits

- Promotes deep relaxation
- Anatomically neutral position, allows for blood and oxygen to flow freely, without restriction
- Calms and focuses the mind

Lie on your back. Feet are relaxed, heels touching, toes fall to the side. Arms are down, alongside the body, close but not touching. Hands turned, with palms facing up to the ceiling. Chin is slightly tucked, extending back of the neck against the mat. Relax your jaw. Place the tip of your tongue behind the top of your two front teeth. This relaxes your jaw, relaxes your tongue and relaxes your optic nerve. Let your belly go soft. Feel it gently rise as you inhale and your lungs inflate. Allow it to softly settle back toward your spine as the air goes out of your lungs.

Try not to control your breathing. Turn your attention to the breath and follow it with your mind. Occupy the mind with the breath. Make the commitment to lying perfectly still while you breath. Start with one minute, just sixty seconds. Watch what happens in your mind as you attempt to be still. Inevitably an imperative urge will arise. Maybe to fix your hair or scratch your nose. Try to create separation between the thought and the action between the impulse and the movement. In this separation is the essence of stillness. This is a practice. If you move, it is not a failure. It is like falling out of a balancing posture. Just get back in. Go back to your commitment to practicing stillness.

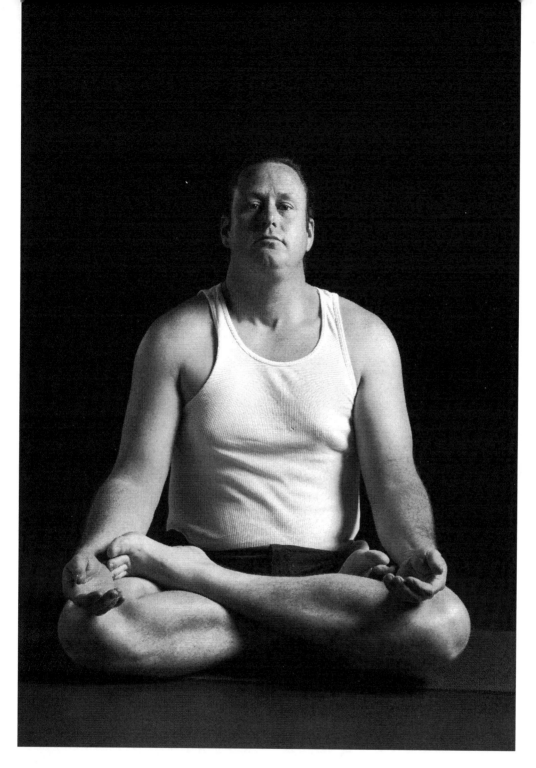

Lotus

Physical Benefits

- Improves sciatica
- Improves digestion
- Strengthens nervous system

Some people prefer to meditate in an upright position. Give Lotus a try, but don't force yourself to sit in an uncomfortable position. There are a multitude of mudras (hand positions). All of these have meaning and subtle effects on your being. Take a little time to research and experiment. Find one that works for you or develop a repertoire so you can match your mudra to your mood.

Sit on the ground. Bend both knees. Pick up right foot and place it on the left thigh. Then pick up the left foot and place it on the right thigh. This requires a great deal of ankle and hip flexibility. You can work up to it slowly.

If the stretch is too intense, do half lotus. You curl one leg underneath and place the top leg in lotus one leg in lotus. Hands rest on knees.

Double Savasana

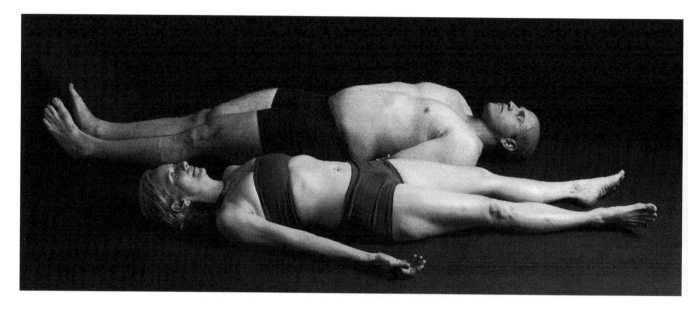

Lie side by side, facing opposite directions. Follow individual instructions for Savasana. You may want to touch the inside hands. Expand the sphere of your awareness to include the person by your side. See if you can feel their breath as it enters and leaves their body. Connect with that which is breathing you.

> It can be very interesting to meditate with a partner. Both Savasanah and Lotus can be performed in pairs.

Physical Benefits

- Same as for single poses, except that you have someone to share them with.

Double Lotus

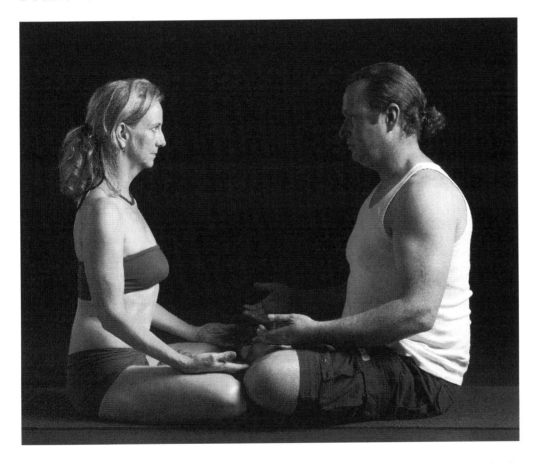

Sit in Lotus facing each other. Knees can be touching or not. Hands can be in mudra or clasped together in front of the hearts. You can choose the degree of contact and connection you are willing to allow.

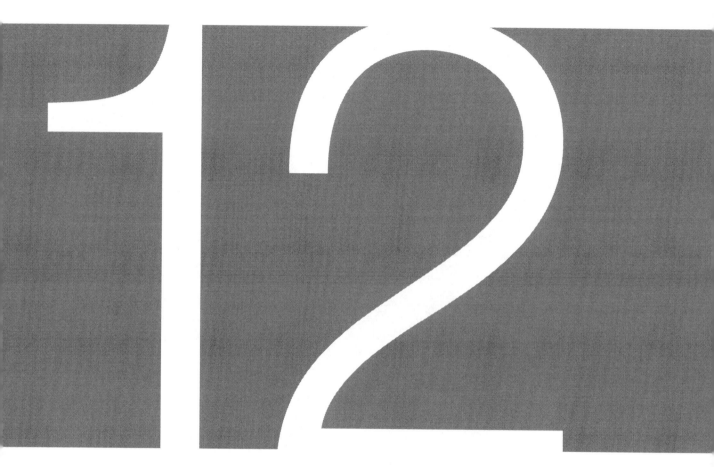

STEP TWELVE

Spiritual Awakening & Giving it Away

- Bridge
- Wheel
- Falcon

"Having had a spiritual awakening as a result of these steps, we tried to carry this message to alcoholics and to practice these principles in all our affairs."

All of these postures are about expanding the chest and opening the heart. This creates more room for blood, air, energy, and love. They can also be a lot of fun. You have worked really hard to get here and should be able to enjoy the fruits of your labor. With the exception of Bridge, these are all advanced postures and should be practiced with care and attention. Moving into advanced poses makes sense when you have reached Step 12. You have developed the strength and skill you need and are ready to move forward into bigger and better things. You have also been sober long enough to have learned how to have fun in sobriety. Relax and enjoy!

Working the 12th step requires you to give it away. You cannot give anything away unless others want what you have. If you have arrived at the last step with a closed heart and unhappy mind, it is unlikely that anyone will ask what you did to get there. By practicing yoga, working the steps and learning to open your heart, you will become much more spiritually fit. Spiritual fitness includes joy. There are times in yoga when I touch joy, or bliss, or whatever that cosmic energy is that bubbles out of the heart and completely absorbs the mind. All of the postures for the 12th step should help you to move in the direction of joy.

Bridge *Seta Bandha Savangasana*

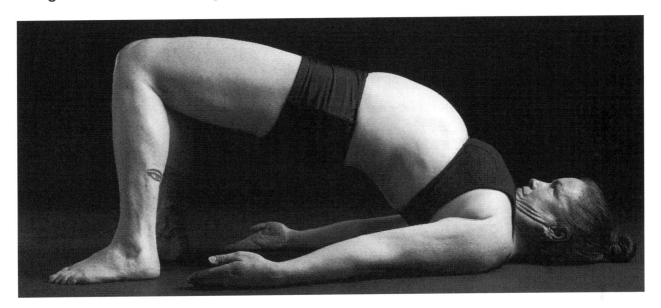

Lie on your back with knees bent. Feet should be firmly planted, directly under knees. Arms are down, alongside body. Inhale deeply, as you exhale, lift hips up. Contract buttocks and press pelvis toward ceiling. Draw chest toward chin. Do not pull chin to chest. To roll down, release neck first and move down along spine to buttocks.

Physical Benefits

- Stretches chest, neck, and spine
- Stimulates abdominal organs
- Opens up lower part of the lungs

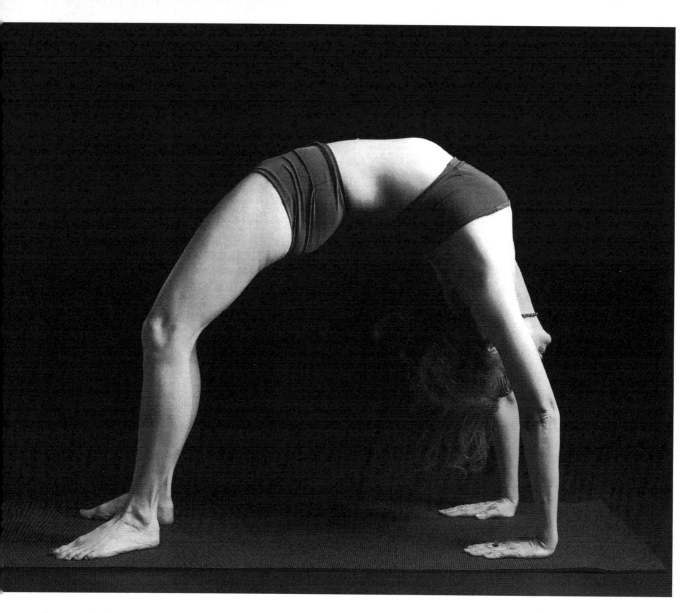

Wheel *Chakra Asana*

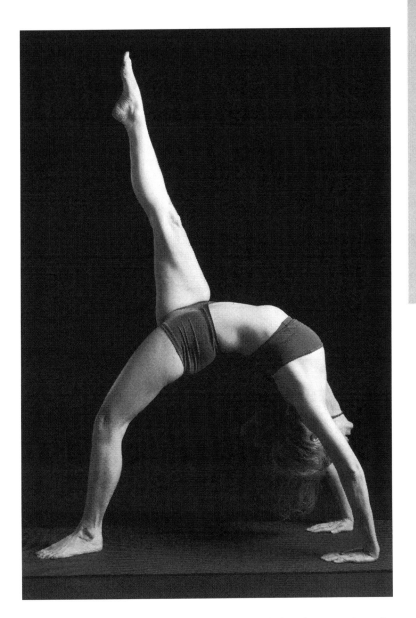

Physical Benefits

- Strengthens hands, arms and legs
- Stretches abdominal muscles
- Stimulates pituitary and thyroid glands

Lie flat on your back. Bend knees and bring feet as close to the buttocks as possible. Keep soles of feet flat on floor. Bend arms and place hands flat on floor directly under each shoulder with fingers pointing back. Hands and feet press against floor, as you arch your spine and lift hips up to the ceiling. You are coming up in to a backbend. Drop head, close your mouth and breathe. To increase the difficulty, lift one leg. Point toes to ceiling. Balance and breathe.

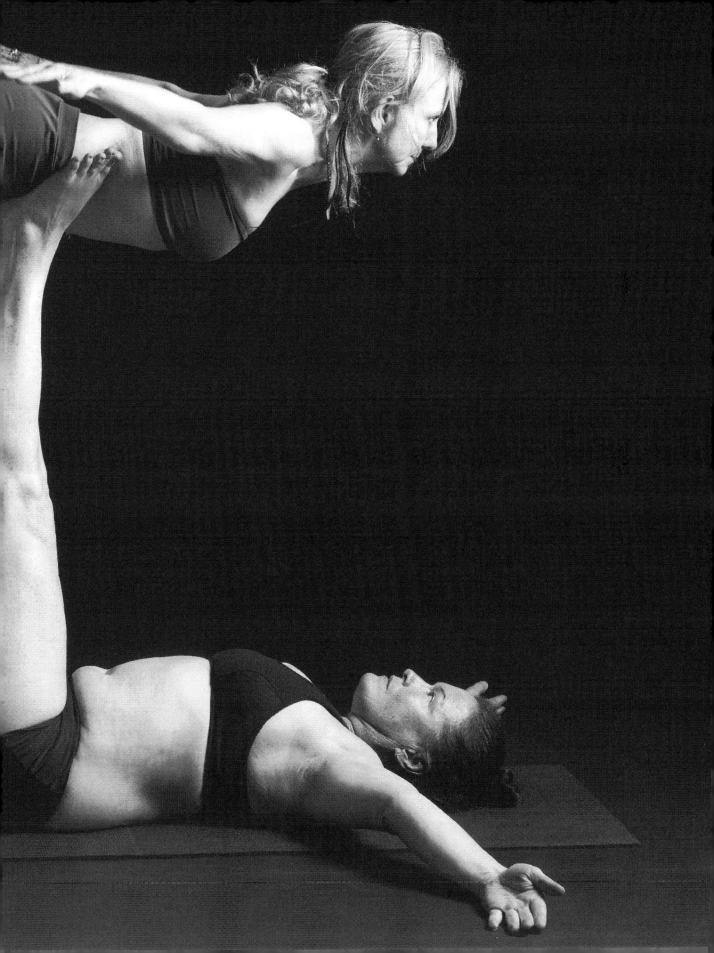

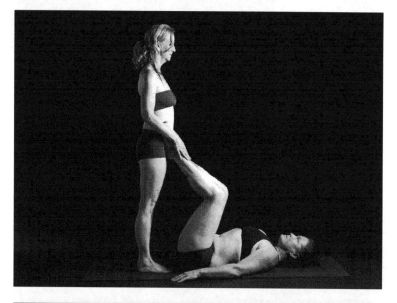

Falcon

As I wrote earlier, lifts can be risky. They are often tricky, especially in the beginning. Always practice in a clear, open space with a soft surface for landing. Be prepared to fall. Falling is part of the process.

Important: Lifts are contraindicated for people with spinal or neck injuries, high blood pressure, a history of strokes and women who are pregnant.

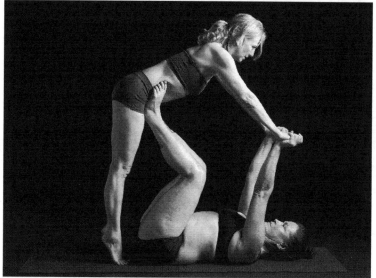

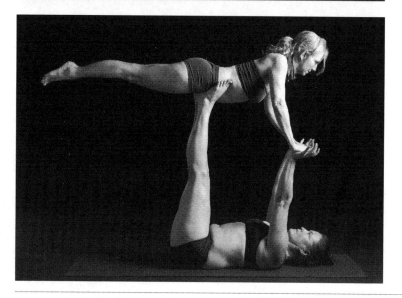

BASIC LIFT

Partner 1 lies on back, pressing lower back onto the mat. Partner 1 bends knees and lifts feet off the floor. Partner 2 stands in front of Partner 1, placing hips on the lifted feet. Partner 2 leans forward, releasing a portion of body weight onto Partner 1's feet. Both partners extend arms toward each other and touch hands, palms flat. This is the foundation of the lift.

Once the foundation is stable, Partner 2 takes small steps forward, continuing to lean more weight into Partner 1's feet. Partner 1 allows knees to bend and thighs to move back toward the chest. Eventually, Partner 1's feet line up over hips. Once you have achieved this alignment, Partner 1 begins to straighten knees and lift Partner 2 off the ground.

Once Partner 1 has legs comfortably straight, check to make sure feet are directly over hips. Arms are straight and lined up with hands right above shoulders.

FALCON

Once you have attained the Basic Lift you can attempt Falcon. Once again, be prepared to fail. Make sure you have a soft place to fall and the skill to roll out safely when you hit the floor.

Partners release hands. Partner 1 brings arms downside and relaxes them. Partner 2 lifts arms up and back, arching from lower spine. Partner 2 pulls shoulders back, extends arms, stretches fingers and finds balance. Switch and repeat.

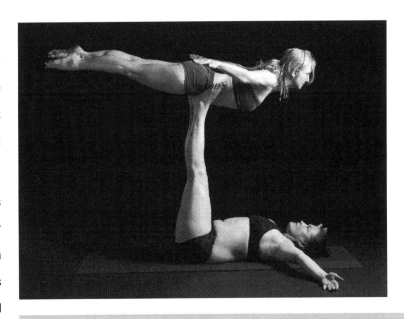

Physical Benefits

PARTNER 1

- Strengthens legs
- Stretches calves and hamstrings
- Develops concentration

PARTNER 2

- Strengthens back and buttocks
- Opens heart and throat chakras
- Induces feelings of flying, freedom, and fearlessness

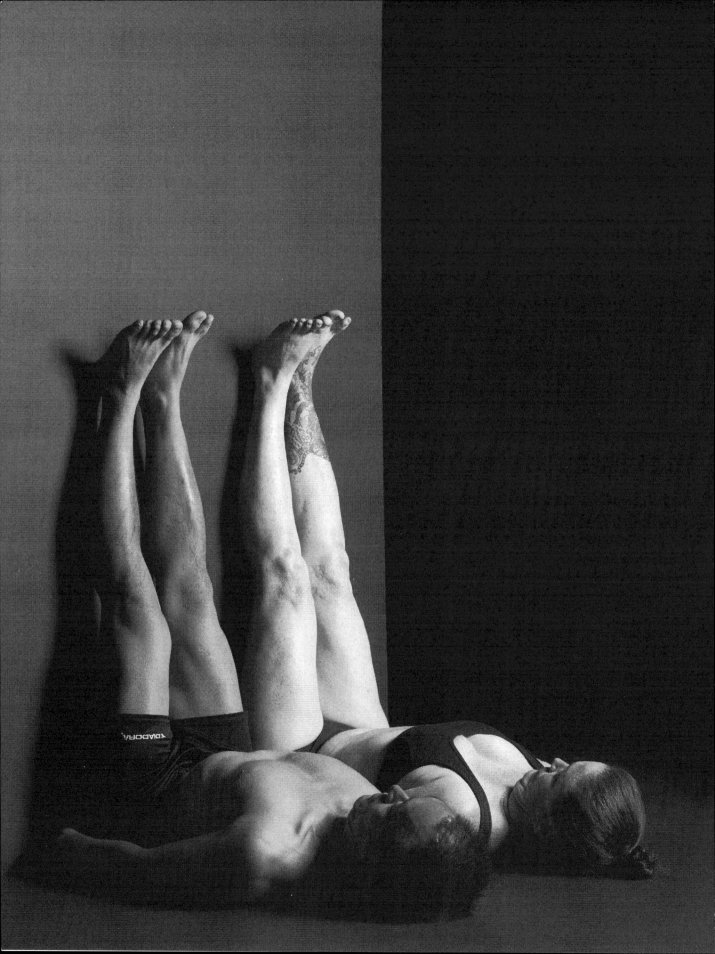

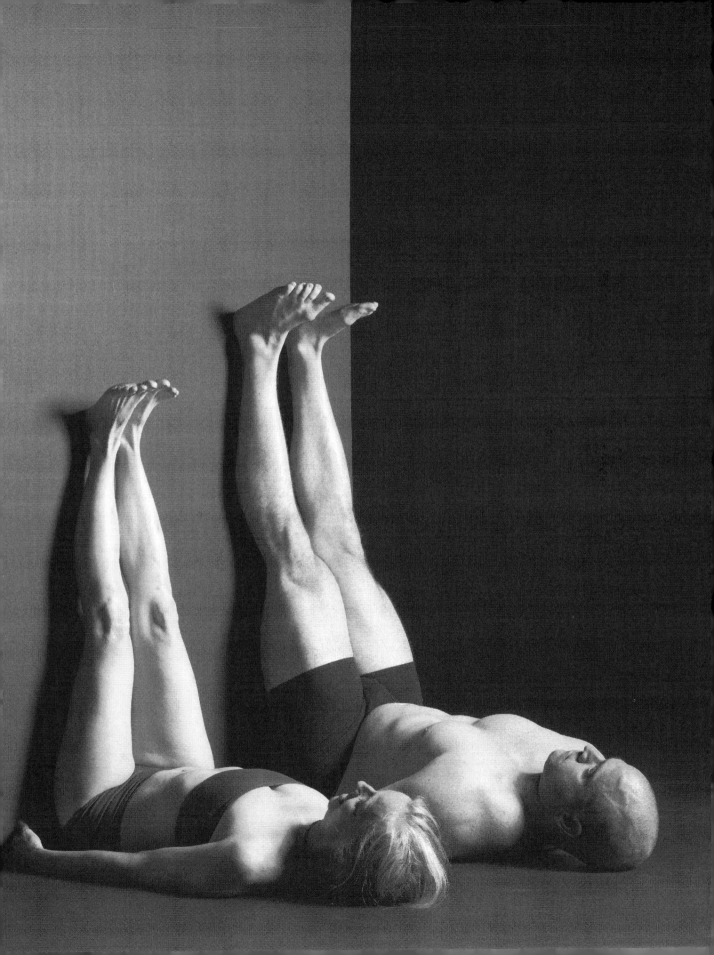

Flows

Working with people in recovery, three of the most common complaints I hear of are depression, anxiety and insomnia. I have put together simple flows of postures that are helpful for these conditions. These are a series of postures you do one after another in the order given. Or, you can pick and choose. Using these asana suggestions as a starting point, you can create your own practice.

Flow I: Anxiety
Flow II: Depression
Flow III: Insomnia

Flow I: Anxiety

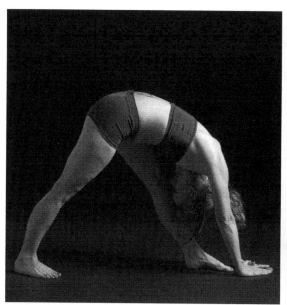

1. Standing Separate Head to Knee

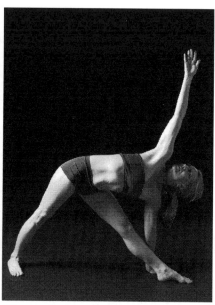

2. Revolved Triangle

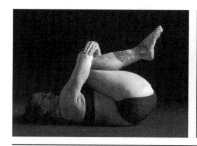

5. Wind Removing

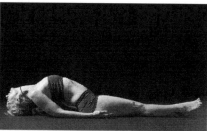

6. Fish

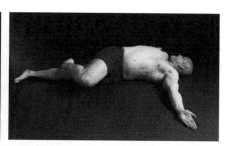

7. Crocodile

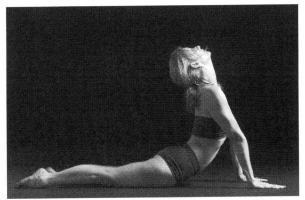
3. Cobra

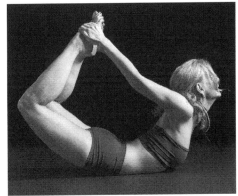
4. Bow

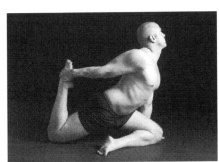
8. Pigeon

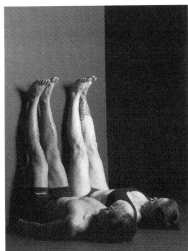
9. Legs up the Wall

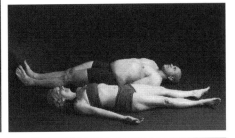
10. Savasana

Flow II: Depression

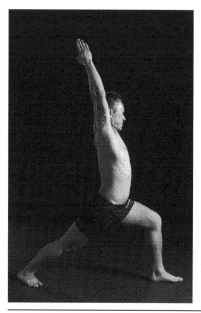
1. Warrior I

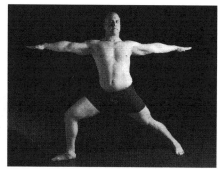
2. Warrior II

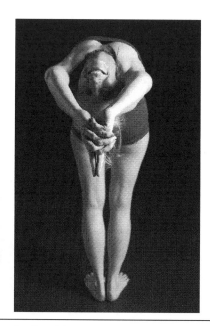
3. Backbend

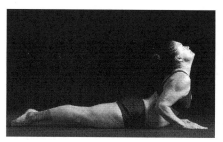
6. Cobra

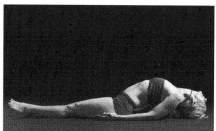
7. Fish

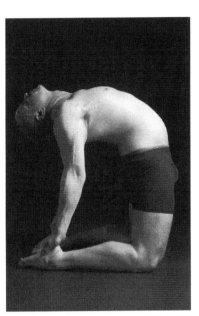
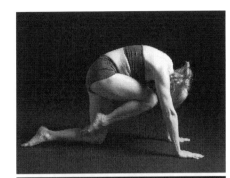
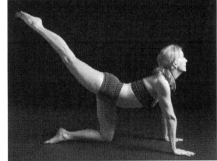

4. Camel

5. Tiger

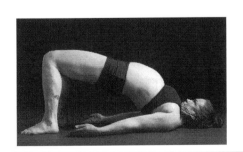
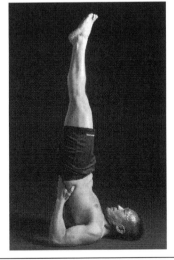
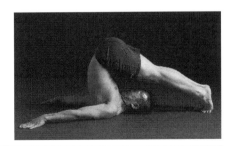

8. Bridge

9. Shoulder Stand

10. Plough

Flow III: Insomnia

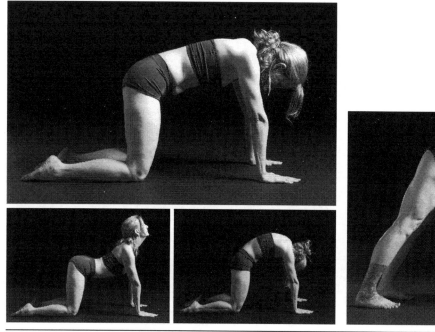

1. Cat / Cow

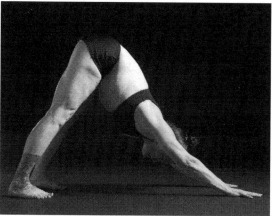

2. Downward Dog

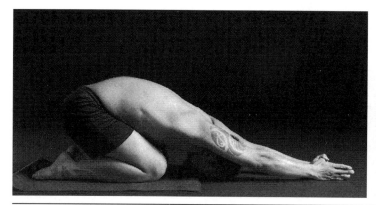

5. Half Tortoise

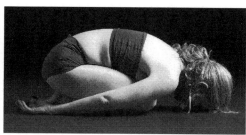

6. Child

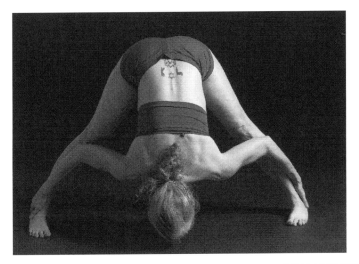
3. Standing Separate Leg Stretching

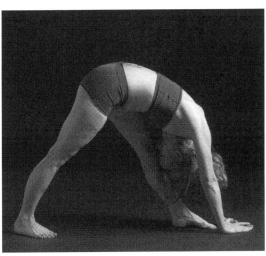
4. Standing Separate Leg Head to Knee

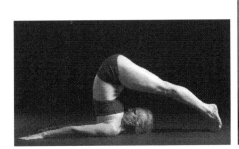
7. Plough

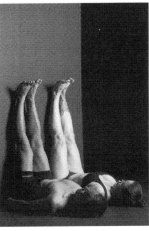
8. Legs up the Wall

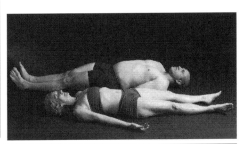
9. Savasana

RECOMMENDED READING

Mark Whitwell
- *Yoga Of Heart: The Healing Power Of Intimate Connection.* Lantern Books, 2004.
- *The Promise: The Secret to Love Sex Intimacy.* Atria, 2010.

Bikram Choudhury
- *Bikram Yoga.* Penguin, 2007.
- *Bikram's Beginning Yoga Class.* Penguin, 2000.

Cain Carroll and Lori Kimata
- *Partner Yoga: Making Contact for Physical, Emotional and Spiritual Growth.* St. Martin's Press, 2000.

Jon Plantania, PhD
- *The 12 Step Restorative Yoga Workbook.* Createspace, 2008.

Alcoholics Anonymous
- *Big Book of Alcoholics Anonymous.* AA World Services Inc., 1976.
- *Twelve Steps and Twelve Traditions.* AA World Services Inc., 1981.
- *Living Sober.* AA World Services Inc., 1975.

Narcotics Anonymous
- *Big Book of Narcotics Anonymous.* NA World Services Inc., 1989.
- *How it Works and Why.* NA World Services Inc., 1993.

Paramahansa Yogananda
- *Autobiography of a Yogi.* Self Realization Fellowship, 1946.

RECOMMENDED READING (continued)

Ram Dass

- *Remember, Be Here Now.* Hanuman Foundation, 1978.
- *Be Love Now (with Rameshwar Das).* Harper Collins, 2010.
- *Journey and Awakening a Meditation Guidebook.* Bantam Books, 1991.

Geshe Michael Roche

- *The Tibetan Book of Yoga.* Doubleday, 2003.

Kevin Griffin

- *One Breath at a Time.* Rodale, 2004.

Swami Prabhavananda with Christopher Isherwood

- *Bhagavad Gita.* Vedanta Press, 1944.

Peter Levine

- *Waking the Tiger: Healing Trauma.* North Atlantic Books, 1997.

David Emerson and Elizabeth Hopper, PhD

- *Overcoming Trauma through Yoga: Reclaiming Your Body.* North Atlantic Books, 2011.

INDEX

A

Abdominal muscles 43, 47, 66, 68, 126

Abdominal organs 30, 74, 82, 102, 124

Acetylcholine 24, 25

Adrenal glands 110

Alternate Nostril Breathing 25

Ankles 32, 54, 56, 92, 106

Anxiety 135-136

Ardha Kurmasana 45-46

Ardha Matsendrasana 70-72

Ardho Mukhe Svanasana 79-80, 139

Arms 42, 66, 76, 80, 126

Assisted Handstand 75-76

B

Back 40, 42, 46, 108, 130

Backbend 39-40, 42, 137

Backpack 67-68

Baddha Konasana 29-30

Bhagavad Gita 8

Balance 47, 66, 92, 108

Balancing Stick 95-98

Basic Lift 49-50, 129-130

Blood flow 46, 50, 56, 68, 82, 110

Bound Angle 29-30

Bow 136

Brain 46, 76

Breathe with Me 57-58

Breathing 22-25

Bridge 124. 138

Buttocks 40, 66, 90, 98, 130

INDEX (continued)

C

Cat/Cow 139

Calves 50, 54, 56, 80, 130

Camel 81-82, 138

Central nervous system 71

Chair 55-56

Chakra Asana 125-126

Chakras 42, 81

Chest 34, 54, 64, 68, 124

Child 33-34, 139

Child/Fish 33-34

Child/Half Tortoise 33-34

Cobra 136, 137

Concentration 47, 50, 66, 92, 108, 130

Cosmic consciousness 21

Crocodile 135

D

Dandayamana-Danurasana 64-66

Dandayamana-Janushirasana 47-48

Depression 137-138

Digestion 46, 90

Dopamine 23

Double Lotus 120

Double Savasana 119

Double Tree 92-93

Double Triangle 109-110

Downward Dog 79-80, 139

E

Eagle 107-108

Ego 48

Eka Pada Kapotasana 99-100

Energy 68, 76

F

Face 50, 64

Falcon 127-130

Fish 135, 137

Fixed Firm 31-32

Flat feet 30

G

Garasana 107-108

Groin 30, 100

H

Halasana 73-74

Half Tortoise 45-46

Hamstrings 50, 80, 130

Hands 126

Hanging Lift 50

Head 50, 68

Head Ache 74

Honoring 83-84

Hips 32, 34, 38, 46, 54, 56, 71, 92, 98, 100, 106

Heart 12-13, 123

Heart Chakra 42, 81, 130

INDEX (continued)

I

Insomnia 139-140

J

Jaw 64

Joints 108

K

Kidneys 102, 110

Knees 32, 47, 92 106

L

Legs 42, 47, 68, 80, 90, 126, 130

Legs Up the Wall 131-132

Lion 61-64

Lotus 117-118

Lower back 34

Lungs 24, 54, 66, 124

M

Mark Whitwell 1-2, 7, 12-13

Massage Table 41-42

Mayan Prayer 114

Meditation 113, 115, 119-120

Metabolism 88

N

Neck 50, 64, 124

Nerves 124

Nitric Oxide 23

O

Optic nerve 64

P

Parathyroid gland 82, 88

Pain tolerance 32

Parasympathetic nervous system 15

Partner postures 18-19, 33-34, 41-42, 49-50, 57-58, 67-68, 75-76, 83-84, 91-92, 101-102, 119-120

Pigeon 99-100

Pituitary gland 76, 126

Plough 73-74, 138, 140

Pranayama 23

Psoas muscle 100

R

Rabbit 87-88

Ram Dass 113

Relaxation 116

Revolved Triangle 135

Rhythmic Breathing 24

INDEX (continued)

S

Sasangasana 87-88

Savasana 115-116

Sciatica 118

Seratonin 23

Seta Bandha Sarvangasana 124-125

Shoulders 40, 42, 50, 54, 97, 109

Shoulder Stand 73-74, 138

Simhasana 61-64

Spine 34, 40, 50, 68, 72-73. 82, 88 , 108, 124

Spinal nerves 90, 110

Spinal Twist 71-72

Standing Bow 65-66

Standing Head to Knee 47-48

Standing Separate Leg Head to Knee 135, 140

Standing Separate Leg Stretching 140

Standing Twist 101-102

Stress 15

Stress response 15

Stomach 71

Stomach muscles 68

Supta Vagrasana 31-32

Sympathetic nervous system 14-15

Synapses 23

T

Thighs 30, 38, 40, 47, 50, 71

Throat 34, 82

Throat Chakra 42, 130

Thyroid gland 74, 82, 88, 126

Tiger 89-90, 138

Tongue 64

Touch 18-19

Trauma 13

Tree 105-106

Triangle 37-38

Trikonasana 37-38

U

Upper arm 56, 98

Urinary tract 100

Ustrasana 81-82

Utkatasana 55-56

V

Vagus nerve 23-24

Vertebra 88

Virabhadrasana 53-54, 137

Vrikasana 105-106

Vygahnasana 89-90

W

Waist 38

Warrior I 53-54, 137

Warrior II 137

Wheel 125-1126

Wind Removing 135

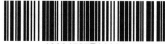

Made in the USA
Middletown, DE
22 July 2017